DATE		

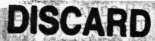

VGM Opportunities Series

OPPORTUNITIES IN MEDICAL TECHNOLOGY CAREERS

Karen Karni
Jane Sidney Oliver

Foreword by
Sharon Zablotney, Ph.D., CLS
President
American Society for Medical Technology

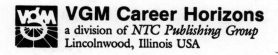

VGM Career Horizons
a division of *NTC Publishing Group*
Lincolnwood, Illinois USA

Cover Photo Credits:
Front cover: upper left and upper
right, photos by Karen Karni;
lower left, Coyahoga Community
College photo; lower right,
AMGen photo.
Back cover: upper left, upper
right, and lower right, photos
by Karen Karni; lower left, U.S.
Department of Public Health
photo.

Library of Congress Cataloging-in-Publication Data

Karni, Karen R.
   Opportunities in medical technology careers / Karen Karni, Jane
Sydney Oliver.

      p.   cm. — (VGM opportunities series)
   Includes bibliographical references.
   ISBN 0-8442-8671-0 : $11.95. — ISBN 0-8442-8672-9 (pbk.) : $8.95
   1. Medical laboratory technology—Vocational guidance.
   I. Oliver, Sydney, 1945– .   II. Title.   III. Series.
   RB37.6.K37   1989
   61D 69'5–dc20
                                                                89-22694
                                                                CIP

Published by VGM Career Horizons, a division of NTC Publishing Group.
© 1990 by NTC Publishing Group, 4255 West Touhy Avenue,
Lincolnwood (Chicago), Illinois 60646-1975 U.S.A.

ABOUT THE AUTHORS

Karen Karni is the Director of the Division of Medical Techology, University of Minnesota Medical School. She has authored numerous articles in education and management in laboratory science, and she is the senior editor of the text, *Clinical Laboratory Management: A Guide for Clinical Laboratory Scientists*.

Dr. Karni has been active in the American Society for Medical Technology (ASMT) and has received several awards from this association: the Sherwood Professional Achievement Award in Education, Immunology Scientific Assembly Award, Scientific Creativity Award, and the Kleiner Award for excellence in writing in the *American Journal of Medical Technology*. She has presented over seventy workshops nationally and internationally and is currently serving as the consulting editor for the Education "In Practice" section of *Clinical Laboratory Science*. She is a former president of the Minnesota Society for Medical Technology and the National Certification Agency for Medical Laboratory Personnel.

Karen Karni worked as a short-term consultant for Project HOPE in Panama, helping to re-establish the medical technology program at the University of Panama. She has also represented the Committee on Allied Health Education and Accreditation (CAHEA) in evaluating the medical laboratory technology program at Kuwait University.

Dr. Karni received her B.S. degree in medical technology from the University of Minnesota and an Ed.M. degree from the State University of New York at Buffalo. She earned a Ph.D. in education from the University of Minnesota.

Jane Sidney Oliver served as professional staff member of the American Society for Medical Technology (ASMT) between 1980 and 1989. Between 1985 and 1988, she served ASMT as Director of Government and Professional Affairs and received the Society's coveted Robin H. Mendelsohn Award for her service in that role. In 1988, she assumed direction of ASMT's Division of Professional Affairs, where she was responsible for managing ASMT's public and media relations, special research projects, membership development, and membership communications. Currently, she is an independent writer in Washington, D.C.

Ms. Oliver's publications include articles and essays which have appeared in such periodicals as the *Journal of Medical Technology,* the *Journal of the American Medical Writers' Association, Association Management,* and *quest: a feminist quarterly.* She coauthored a chapter on clinical laboratory scientists'roles as consultants to physicians operating office laboratories in *Clinical Laboratory Science: Strategies for Practice* (1989) and a pioneering monograph on the quality of services and the evolution of practice in physician office laboratories.

Ms. Oliver received her baccalaureate degree in English literature, with a minor in political science, from the University of Tennessee, in Knoxville, in 1967. She received her master of arts degree in English in 1969, also from the University of Tennessee.

ACKNOWLEDGMENTS

The success of every book is the result of collective effort, but its shortcomings belong to the authors alone. We express deep appreciation to the following colleagues for their encouragement and assistance: Lucy Randles, Douglas Estry, Kathryn Doig, Patricia Ziemer, Pat Solberg, Elaine Sommers, Janice Putnam, Leanna Lindquist, John Fauser, Barbara Weithaus, Lisa Creeden, Captain Danny Seanger (U.S. Air Force), Colonel James E. Spiker (U.S. Army), and Captain Roy Koehn (U.S. Navy).

We also appreciate the staff assistance of Carol El Ghandour, Lillian Sarkinen, and Laura Walker. Special thanks to Catherine Meschter and Michael, Erik, and Jake Karni for their patience and faith.

We are also grateful to the American Society for Medical Technology for its cooperation in furnishing essential references cited in this text and for general support and encouragement for the project and its authors.

FOREWORD

Clinical laboratory science careers are exciting, challenging, and rewarding. Karen Karni and Jane Sidney Oliver have captured the spirit of this excitement in this book through their description of the profession and its many career opportunities. If you are searching for a health care career that will give you an opportunity to apply your intellectual abilities, help other people, and interact with other dynamic professionals, then a career in clinical laboratory science will interest you.

The constant change being experienced in health care today is reflected in the clinical laboratory. New technologies, changing professional roles, and alternate health care delivery sites all create the dynamic environment in which laboratorians work. This degree of change opens doors of opportunity through which laboratorians are reaching new heights of professional endeavors. They find themselves on the frontiers of health care, isolating probes to detect genetic errors, formulating diagnostic algorithms to aid physicians in their laboratory diagnosis, or consulting with other health care professionals. In each of these roles the laboratorian will draw upon her or his knowledge of science, skills of communication, and analytic and problem-solving abilities.

As you read this book, the vastness of the field of clinical laboratory science will be revealed to you again and again. There will be an opportunity for you to analyze your interests and skills and to match them with those needed by laboratory professionals. Sample high school and college curricula are included to guide you in your selection of your course of study. This is an exciting time for you, an opportunity to fulfill your goals through a rewarding career as a clinical laboratory professional.

Sharon L. Zablotney, Ph.D., CLS
President
American Society for Medical Technology

PREFACE

This book provides a description of the career opportunities afforded to men and women by the profession of clinical laboratory science. Those interested in science, in laboratory work, in interacting with people, in serving the community and contributing to the betterment of humankind will do well to consider this profession as a career choice.

The profession of clinical laboratory science has evolved since the early 1900s. Presently there are an estimated 250,000 laboratory personnel in the United States, the majority (160,000) being clinical laboratory scientists educated at the baccalaureate level. This book is intended to encourage students to complete this kind and level of education. However, job descriptions of other major laboratory personnel are provided within the book as well.

The terminology in laboratory science is changing. In the past, the title "medical technologist" was used to denote a graduate of a baccalaureate program in laboratory science. Now, the title "clinical laboratory scientist" is being used with increasing frequency. In this book, both titles may be found. For example, the accrediting agency, the National Accrediting Agency for Clinical Laboratory Sciences (NAACLS) uses the new title, as does the certification designation, "clinical laboratory scientist" granted by the National Certification Agency. However, the Committee on Allied Health Education and Accreditation lists accredited programs under the title "medical technologist." We support the terminology of "clinical laboratory science," since it more accurately describes this profession.

Everyone is ultimately confronted with the decision of selecting a career. There are those rare individuals who early in life know what they wish to do and pursue that career unwaveringly. However, most of us are not that single-minded. Indeed, this book is to help those who may be uncommitted, to decide whether this profession meets their expectations, interests, and abilities.

One inevitably asks "How can I tell if I am the kind of person who will be a successful professional in this field?" Two factors have the greatest influence upon the answer: motivation and ability. The first might be evaluated by how much an individual finds out about a profession of interest, through reading, interviews, tours, and volunteer work. The second can be somewhat evaluated by a review of a high school or college transcript. Both, however, are crucial to the success one has in reaching a goal.

Through this book, then, we hope to entice men and women to join our ranks. Clinical laboratory science offers many job opportunities. It also provides satisfaction in work done well. Finally, it represents science at the "cutting edge," as new technologies make this profession more exciting, more intricate, and more needed.

INTRODUCTION

WHAT DOES A LABORATORY PROFESSIONAL DO?

You look closely through a microscope to examine the specimen. Separate its components. Freeze it. Stain it with different solutions. Magnify it. Whirl it. Add reagents to it. Determine its endpoints—qualitative, quantitative. With precision. With accuracy. With speed.

It takes intelligence, discipline, a positive attitude.

You have to want to work with both your mind and your hands. To like biology and chemistry. To use microscopes, simple and complicated instruments, computers.

There are challenges: to master new principles, techniques, methodologies. To provide needed information. To experiment. To devise new ways of testing. To perform sophisticated procedures, sometimes under pressure of time and in life or death situations.

And there is satisfaction; demonstrating competence in performing well. Being productive in a concrete way. Providing quality service. Working with colleagues. And, most of all, knowing you have a vital part in the diagnosis, treatment, and care of your fellow human beings.

CONTENTS

Overview. What is medical technology? Definitions of
medical technology. Changes in the field. Employment
outlook. Salaries outlook. Job satisfaction. Financial
requirements. Conclusion.

Overview. Laboratory distribution. Laboratory settings.
Advantages and disadvantages of working in various
laboratory settings. Laboratory safety. Summary.

Pathologist. Medical technologist (clinical laboratory
scientist). Cytotechnologist. Medical (clinical) laboratory
technician. Other laboratory personnel. Practitioner
attributes. Summary.

CHAPTER 1

THE SCOPE AND PRACTICE OF MEDICAL TECHNOLOGY

OVERVIEW

Medical technology, or clinical laboratory science, takes its practitioners on a fascinating journey to the very center of life, to the heart of the age-old mysteries of disease and good health.

Using complex, computer-aided technologies, precision electronic instruments, high-powered microscopes, and the most basic human senses, medical technology professionals draw on medicine, the social and biological sciences, computer science, and communications in their roles as information specialists in the laboratory, the "control room" of modern health care.

Medical technology is also a rapidly evolving industry of major proportions. In the United States alone, we spend some $20 billion each year for tests performed in over 100,000 clinical laboratories.

Typically, through detailed microscopic, chemical, or visual analysis of specimens taken from body substances, clinical laboratory scientists (sometimes called medical technologists) identify, verify, and report the presence or absence of chemicals, microorganisms, enzymes, proteins, and other substances, and the composition and function of cells, tissues, and organs. The six billion tests they perform each year help physicians diagnose diseases, determine their causes, prescribe correct treatment, prevent unwelcome drug interactions, discover substance abuse or other impairments, and perhaps most important, promote good health.

Clinical laboratory scientists and other laboratory practitioners are found throughout the health care delivery system, as well as in numerous other settings. Those who choose to work in the clinical laboratory practice in hospitals, independent commercial laboratories, clinics, doctors' offices, Red Cross and other blood banks, public health departments, ambulatory care centers, and other such settings. Some work abroad, in the Peace Corps or Project Hope, or in private or government facilities in other countries.

Most professionals work in clinical laboratories performing the analytical procedures just described. Many others, however, provide specialized services in a variety of essential health care roles, often in hospitals but also in other health care delivery settings. Some, for example, ensure the quality of the nation's supply of blood and blood products used for transfusions in surgery, postoperatively, and for other needs. Others perform tissue and cell analyses essential for bone marrow, kidney, skin, heart, and other organ transplants. Some put their skills to work for *in vitro* fertilization laboratories where human sperm and ova are joined in an artificial environment outside the living body to remedy sterility. Still others work as researchers in public health departments where they help epidemiologists trace the origin and spread of infectious diseases. And some go on to other roles, serving as hospital infection control officers and as managers in the upper echelons of hospital administration.

These are just a few of the options open to the qualified clinical laboratory professional within health care. Consider also the array of roles outside the health care mainstream such as biogenetics; occupational health; environmental health; independent consulting; education and higher education administration; industrial research, product development, marketing, and sales; and veterinary science and criminology (forensics). Few other fields offer baccalaureate graduates basic preparation for so many possible career paths.

Clinical laboratory science offers the prospective student another important advantage. According to almost all experts, the current shortage of medical technologists is rapidly expanding. That, coupled with increasing demand for clinical laboratory services, means that in almost every area of the country, jobs are and will continue to be plentiful, and salaries and benefits—already reasonably good especially at the starting level—will rise. In fact, in many areas, qualified medical technologists can take their pick of several openings and get additional, attractive bonuses in the bargain.

For bright men and women with sound backgrounds in the natural sciences who are attracted to biology, technology, problem solving, and helping people, this profession offers many satisfying career options and an enviable degree of job security.

WHAT IS MEDICAL TECHNOLOGY?

Probably no other profession is both so important to health care, and yet so little known (and confusing to those outside the field) as is medical technology. Because clinical laboratory professionals historically have had somewhat limited contact with patients, most people know less about them than about the other health care workers we do have contact with. And yet, the information the clinical laboratory professional provides is largely responsible for the appropriateness of the care provided by nurses, family physicians, surgeons and other doctors, pharmacists, therapists, and other health professionals. Each of them relies in part on laboratory data to help plan or implement the course of treatment that is just right for each patient.

At the same time, few fields in all of health care are as confusing for those outside the profession as is medical technology. There are many reasons for the confusion. First, clinical laboratory practitioners (the term used here for all levels of practice) are known by a bewildering number of professional titles. Second, they work in a huge number and variety of settings. Third, there are differences even within the profession about what various clinical laboratory practitioners should be called and what their roles should be.

These facts make the task of counting them all but impossible. Accordingly, no one knows for sure how many individuals the profession comprises. Estimates range from a low of just over a quarter-million to perhaps more than a half-million, and might soar higher still, depending upon who is counting and whether those who have pursued a nonclinical career (such as teaching, industrial reasearch and development, or marketing and sales, for instance) are included.

DEFINITIONS OF MEDICAL TECHNOLOGY

To begin to understand this complex field, it helps to remember that medical technologists assume many roles within and outside of the health service delivery system.

It might also be helpful to remember that because the field is constantly changing (in response to new technologies, health care cost-containment pressures, and variations in health care needs), new roles for medical technologists are being created every year.

The American Society for Medical Technology (ASMT), the oldest and largest of the professional societies devoted exclusively to clinical laboratory science, summarizes the scope of practice of the profession. (See appendix E.)

Although many definitions exist, in the simplest terms, medical technology is the profession concerned with providing information based on the performance of analytical tests upon human body substances to detect evidence of or to prevent disease or impairment, and to promote and monitor good health.

Among the thousands of complex and routine tests available are many well known to most people. Almost everyone has had at least one complete blood count (CBC) performed to detect blood disorders such as anemia or leukemia, or a urinalysis used to screen for numerous conditions. Most of us have had our blood typed and tested for compatibility, so that when we donate or receive blood, we and others are ensured of a safe, effective transfusion. More and more of us are having our cholesterol levels checked, to lessen the risk of heart disease. Some of us monitor our blood sugar levels to correct conditions like hypoglycemia and treat diseases like diabetes. Other well-known clinical laboratory tests include premarital tests, pregnancy tests, antibody tests for immunological disease, throat cultures for infections, and tests for alcohol or drug levels.

The simple definition of medical technology just provided focused exclusively on the laboratory information function these practitioners provide, that is, on clinical practice. A better definition takes into account the important fact that since its origins (see chapter 7 for a brief history), the field has grown in complexity and responsibility from an ancillary, or helping, occupation limited to elementary functions, to its status today as a multifacted profession that includes clinical practice and many other roles as well.

A more accurate definition, then, might read as follows:

> Clinical laboratory professionals assume many roles within and out- side health services delivery. In traditional laboratory service delivery they provide essential clinical information based on performing and ensuring the quality of tests of human body fluids and other substances. Integral parts of their responsibility are verifying, interpreting, and reporting the results of these tests directly to attending physicians. Many also assist physicians in correlating test results with patient data, and recommend tests and test sequences in light of known clinical considera- tions. They also perform a wide range of management and supervisory roles, including serving as clinical laboratory directors, managers of laboratory sections, and supervisors of junior technologists, techni- cians, phlebotomists, and other laboratory practitioners. They are ex- pected to contribute to the body of knowledge comprising the profession. They work in cooperation with pathologists and with other physicians and scientists who specialize in such disciplines as clinical chemistry or microbiology. Their services are essential for preventing, detecting, and diagnosing disease and impairment, and for promoting good health.
>
> Clinical laboratory scientists may also choose among many other roles within the health service delivery system but outside the traditional laboratory, including critical research roles; hospital and other institu- tion management and administration roles; independent consulting; and positions in institutional infection control, public health, and epidemiol- ogy, to name a few.
>
> Those who do not choose careers in health care may choose among education and higher education administration; diagnostic equipment, pharmaceutical and many other types of industrial research and product development, marketing, sales, or product representation; veterinary science; forensics; environmental or occupational safety and health; and many other career paths.

Although clinical laboratory practitioners assist physicians and in the laboratory work closely with and are occasionally supervised by medical specialists called pathologists, medical technology is not part of the practice of medicine. However, because some pathologists provide a few clinical laboratory services (though most are engaged in anatomical laboratory services), and because medical technology has a history closely associated with pathology, some pathologists and others disagree.

Nevertheless, several state attorneys general and the United States Department of Health and Human Services (HHS), in a regulation upheld by the United States Court of Appeals, find that medicine and medical technology are different professions.

In a 1976 opinion, for instance, the Attorney General for Minnesota, Warren Spannaus, wrote to Arthur W. Poore, Executive Secretary, Minnesota Board of Medical Examiners (Correspondence. January 5, 1976 [303c]):

> You ask . . . substantially the following. . . .
>
> Does the scientific testing and reporting of results of medical laboratories of samples obtained from human beings performed only for and at the request of licensed physicians, constitute the practice of medicine?
>
> We answer your question in the negative.
>
> In our opinion, the function performed by the medical laboratories does not constitute diagnosis. . . . Rather, the labs are engaged in ascertaining observable or quantifiable facts. . . .
>
> This result is consistent with the opinions of Attorneys General of other states dealing with the line between the unauthorized practice of medicine and licensed laboratory testing. . . .

CHANGES IN THE FIELD

Few fields are undergoing so much change so quickly as clinical laboratory science. A definition showing the scope of this profession and hinting at this change was offered by a past president of the American Society for Medical Technology in *Shaping the Future of Clinical Laboratory Practice: Proceedings of the Conference.* ASMT, 1986, iii:

The laboratory profession during this conference does not refer to the hospital alone. Even within the hospital it does not refer to the physical space that the laboratory occupies. The laboratory profession encompasses those activities of performing, reporting, interpreting and correlating laboratory tests designed for the promotion of health [and the] prevention and treatment of disease through the application of scientific principles of biology, chemistry, and physics as they relate to [human] physiologic and biochemical processes. The laboratory profession includes a number of defined, specialized areas of competence and also incorporates social science to serve its primary purpose. Further, research, consultation, education and administration are integral features of the profession.

The opening comment that the profession is not bound by the four walls of the laboratory is very important. The reference, of course, is to the very rapid changes the profession is experiencing, even now, as a consequence of new developments in technology.

Three technological developments in particular have already begun to change the profession radically. First, refinements in the microchip have made it possible to store and process huge amounts of information in a very small space. Second, the perfection of dry reagents used in testing have extended the shelf-life of these chemicals, improved their portability, and made them much easier to use. Third, the discovery of the monoclonal antibody that allows clinical laboratory scientists to detect even minute quantities of a specific substance contained in a body specimen has changed the practice of laboratory science.

Collectively, these advances have propelled the manufacture of small, relatively inexpensive desk-top testing instruments and even smaller and cheaper test kits, such as those used in pregnancy testing. In turn, these instruments and kits have made it possible to perform many common tests in doctors' offices and ambulatory care centers, on hospital wards, and even at home, rather than in traditional laboratory settings. Some analysts believe that by the year 2000, every American household will use one or more of these test kits regularly.[1]

---

[1]Gossel, Thomas A. "Home Testing Products for Self-Monitoring." *American Journal of Hospital Pharmacy*, 45 (May 1988): 1119–26.

Test kits, desk-top instruments, and other technological advancements soon to come are changing the nature and expanding the boundaries of traditional medical technology. They are sparking new ideas among educators and managers about the roles the profession should and must take on in tomorrow's laboratory with and without walls. It is too early to say exactly what effects those changes will have on test menus, laboratory personnel, and health services delivery. But change always brings opportunity, and the profession is already considering what new opportunities the future holds.

Principle Practice Areas within the Field

The following principle practice areas within the field are adapted from brief descriptions provided in *Medical Technology Program,* a pamphlet prepared by the Medical Technology Program of the Michigan State University, East Lansing, Michigan:

1. *Clinical chemistry.* Analysis of bodily fluids for elements including glucose, protein, sodium, and cholesterol to detect diseases such as diabetes and heart attacks.
2. *Hematology.* Evaluation of red blood cells, white blood cells, and platelets for diseases like anemia and leukemia.
3. *Hemostasis.* Evaluation of the blood clotting mechanism to detect diseases like hemophilia.
4. *Microbiology.* Identification of bacteria, viruses, fungi, and parasites that cause infections, as well as of the antibiotics that will be effective in treatment.
5. *Urinalysis.* Physical, chemical, and microscopic analysis, which may indicate disease within the urinary tract or other body systems.
6. *Immunohematology.* Performance of blood typing and tests, which provide compatible blood for transfusion; also called blood banking.
7. *Immunology.* Evaluation of the body's immune system to detect diseases of impaired immune function and to ensure the compatibility of organs for transplantation.

EMPLOYMENT OUTLOOK

Most analysts close to the field believe that the serious and growing shortage of qualified personnel and the growing demand for clinical laboratory services create an outstanding employment outlook.

The Bureau of Labor Statistics (BLS) of the U.S. Department of Labor reports that clinical laboratory technologists and technicians held about 239,000 jobs in 1986, and expects employment of clinical laboratory workers to grow about as fast as the average for all occupations through the year 2000. Its projections for year 2000 employment are based on low, moderate, and high economic, labor force, and employment growth assumptions. These translate, respectively, to 285,000 jobs, 296,000 jobs, and 307,000 jobs. On average, the Bureau of Labor Statistics projects 57,000 new jobs in clinical laboratory science by 2000, an increase of twenty-four percent over 1986 rates.

Medical technology is one of a huge group of allied health occupations and professions that (according to the American Society of Allied Health Professions) accounts easily for three million workers, or over half the nation's health work force.

Allied health professionals comprise over two hundred occupations other than medicine, dentistry, pharmacy, and nursing, and they are not necessarily always direct care givers. For example, allied health professions include medical record administrators; physical, occupational, and respiratory therapists; psychologists; audiologists; physician assistants; and medical technologists as well as many others.

In 1988, the Institute of Medicine (IOM) of the National Academy of Sciences published an extensive study of these fields, tellingly titled *Allied Health Services: Avoiding Crises,* because of the Institute's concerns about the growing shortage of allied health personnel. Speaking about *all* allied health fields, the IOM said:

> Barring major economic or health care financing contradictions, growth in the number of jobs for allied health workers will substantially exceed the nation's average rate of growth for all jobs. Unless some existing trends are moderated, the flow of practitioners into the workforce through graduation from education programs will be, at best, stable.

According to the IOM in other words, without significant changes, demand for allied health practitioners will increase faster than the national average for all workers, but at the same time, the supply of new graduate practitioners, even "at best," will remain as it is currently.

For clinical laboratory science specifically, the IOM was more cautious. In the same study it said:

> For . . . other fields, such as clinical laboratory technology . . . there are factors that could cause instability in both supply and demand. For these fields the market is more likely to make the needed adjustments and serious disruptions are less likely to occur.

However, as we show later in this chapter, leading representatives of the medical technology field believe the outlook is much stronger than even the respectable growth anticipated by either the Bureau of Labor Statistics or the Institute of Medicine in their comparatively conservative outlooks.

Factors Affecting Allied Health Employment Predictions

Employment outlooks for most allied health fields, including medical technology, vary considerably from forecaster to forecaster. This is partly due to radical changes in health care economics initiated in 1983, explained later in this chapter (see also chapter 7), and other problems.

Although this is changing, as the IOM noted in *Allied Health Services: Avoiding Crises,* historically there has been "relatively low interest and investment of public resources in learning about the allied health workforce."

Analysts offer many explanations. Some contrast the slim amount of data available about the allied health professions with the wealth of information about medicine. They also explain how low public interest is in the allied health professions partly because of the fact that women predominate in most of them. Others note that many of these fields, like medical technology, are difficult to define. They point to the numerous, often overlapping titles, and to the fact that many fields, including medical technology, are not uniformly licensed and thus lack even the "scope of practice" definitions found in licensure laws for fields like nursing and medicine. Finally, most acknowledge that, where definitions do exist, they: (1) nearly always spark more controversy than agreement; (2) for political or other reasons, might well be too narrow to accurately represent the true range of duties assumed by these practitioners; and (3) given the rapid pace of technological change, are often obsolete almost as soon as written. All these factors make for difficulties in designing and conducting reliable data collection studies.

Outlook for Medical Technology

Despite these weaknesses in data collection, however, even the Institute of Medicine acknowledges, in *Allied Health Services: Avoiding Crises,* that demand for clinical laboratory services could exceed the twenty-four percent growth predicted by the Bureau of Labor Statistics.

That comes closer to the great optimism expressed by most national organizations representing medical technologists. These organizations collect information about their practitioners and otherwise monitor changes the profession is experiencing. Because they are closer than other observers to the day-to-day realities of practice, and because they have so much at stake when occupational forecasts are mistaken, they often make a point of detecting important demographic currents earlier and more accurately.

SUPPLY FACTORS

The supply of qualified personnel has a great deal to do with whether job outlooks are vigorous or not. When supply does not keep up with demand, the employment outlook, of course, favors the job seeker, as is the case now.

Investigations conducted in 1987, 1988, and 1989 by the American Society for Medical Technology (ASMT) and by the American Society of Clinical Pathologists (ASCP) and its Board of Registry suggest that the shortage of clinical laboratory science practitioners is already serious and will worsen.

In a December 1987 poll of its state and territorial chapters, the American Society for Medical Technology found that 62.5 percent reported a shortage of medical technologists; 43 percent reported a shortage of clinical technicians; and 36 percent reported a shortage of phlebotomists. Later data from an unpublished study conducted for ASCP by Market Opinion Research released November 30, 1988, found that 70 percent of all laboratories surveyed reported difficulty filling vacancies at the staff technologist level; 41 percent reported difficulty filling vacancies at the technical level; and 39 percent reported difficulty filling positions at the phlebotomist level. ASCP also indicated 46 percent difficulty filling staff level cytotechnologist positions, and 37 percent difficulty filling staff level histologic technician slots.

Two factors are generally taken to explain the shortage of qualified medical technologists: declining numbers of students entering into and graduating from accredited education programs, and attrition of experienced professionals.

Though there is some debate about cause, several reasons are often cited, most of which pertain to both declining enrollment and attrition as well as to most allied health fields. They include:

1. expanded employment opportunities for women;
2. mistaken employment outlooks dating from 1983;
3. increased competition across all occupations for a declining number of high school graduates;
4. more salary compression in fields within allied health;
5. the comparative low visibility of medical technology as a professional option, contrasted, for instance, with nursing or medicine; and
6. unrealistic perceptions about the risk of exposure to infectious disease.

One explanation sometimes given for the shortage is the rate of closure of medical technology education programs mostly in small hospitals. However, closures have occurred mostly among the small hospital programs, because of the very tight hospital economic climate inaugurated in 1983, and because of declining student enrollment. Therefore, most experts view them as a symptom of the shortage, not a cause.

Changes in the reimbursement of health services to Medicare beneficiaries paid for by the federal government triggered a restructuring particularly in hospitals. That economic tightening also led to overly pessimistic employment scenarios for some allied health fields. Experience has shown that for medical technology, for instance, these forecasts were often seriously mistaken. Nevertheless, they helped to discourage new enrollments into the profession, the effects of which it might still be feeling.

Attrition among experienced professionals from clinical practice to other career paths reportedly occurs for advancement, salary, and other aspirations, and because of the pressures often associated with clinical practice.

Unrealistic perceptions about the risk of infection sometimes are mentioned as a contributor to declining enrollment. Most practitioners, however, are quick to point out that the incidence of accidental exposure to infectious disease is miniscule. They also acknowledge that the laboratory is a controlled environment subject to the most rigorous mandatory and voluntary precautions against exposure, and is experienced in dealing with problem substances.

Increased competition among all science-based professions for a declining number of high school science graduates (thanks partly to the so-called "baby bust") is expected to continue to be a factor in declining enrollments into most allied health professions, including clinical laboratory science.

Finally, thanks to the efforts of feminists and civil rights activists, today there are broader career and job opportunities for women than at any point in history. Significantly, however, career-wide earnings in fields outside allied health are higher than for many allied health fields.

These developments have shrunk and are expected to continue to shrink the supply pool of future allied health practitioners. To the extent that demand and supply influence how the marketplace sets compensation packages (salaries and benefits), and to the extent that current conditions prevail, these factors are expected to greatly increase the likelihood of a favorable employment outlook for clinical laboratory science graduates.

DEMAND

Major factors affecting demand for medical technological services of course also escalate demand for qualified practitioners. These include general population demographics, technological developments, and social developments. According to the Bureau of Labor Statistics:

[c]ontinued expansion of the clinical laboratory field is foreseen for three fundamental reasons. First is the increase in disease and disability that will accompany rapid growth of the middle-aged and older population. Second is the probability of new, more powerful diagnostic tests. Advances in biotechnology have already changed testing methods through the use of monoclonal antibodies and other advanced technologies that permit rapid, simple and accurate testing. As further advances occur, they are likely to spur more testing. And lastly, research laboratories that work to find the cause, treatment and cure for diseases such as acquired immune deficiency syndrome (AIDS) are expanding dramatically in response to increased funding from public and private sources.

The size and composition of the population as a whole has a major effect on demand for health care, and thus the potential to affect the employment outlook significantly. Between 1986 and 2000, the Bureau of the Census predicts a slowing of the growth rate for the American population as a whole, but an increase in the number of people aged sixty-five and over, with a corresponding increase in demand for and intensity of consumption of health care resources.

Other population factors will have an as yet uncertain effect on demand. For instance, the proportion of minorities in the U.S. population will increase by the year 2000. While distressing factors such as diminished financial and geographic access to health care among minorities will have an impact on demand, the higher prevalence among some minorities of chronic diseases especially (such as diabetes and heart disease) will also affect demand.

Technological change—driven by advances discussed earlier and soft technologies such as genetic engineering—is revolutionizing medical technology. Predictions in an article by Mark S. Lifshitz and Robert P. de Cresce, entitled ''The Clinical Lab of the Future,'' *Medical Laboratory Observer,* 20, no. 1 (January 1988), pp. 30–33, are exciting:

Implanted biosensors will give "real-time" health status reports and diminish the lag in results for many tests. Nuclear magnetic resonance will help identify many of numerous compounds; DNA probes and molecular biology will transform how and when diseases and organisms are identified; robots will handle biohazardous materials and repetitive work alike; bar codes will simplify specimen handling from the bedside throughout the laboratory.

These and other expected advancements will not only expand the "menu" of tests available, but probably will also increase the number of tests performed. Technology will have different effects on demand for practitioners at different levels. But if history is any guide, as many jobs will be created as will be taken by automation.

Social developments also have increased demand and, interacting with new technologies, will continue to do so. For instance, changes in attitudes toward drugs and other substances, combined with technological advancements, have helped turn testing for drug use from a relatively minor field into a multi-million dollar industry with still more growth anticipated if legal and ethical questions are satisfactorily resolved. Similarly, the identification of human immunodeficiency virus (HIV) coupled with medical, epidemiological, legal, political, ethical, and other social evaluations of its priority, have made the phrase "AIDS screening tests" a household word. Thanks to advancements in biogenetics, other developments like these will occur with increased demand for medical technological services and qualified practitioners.

OUTLOOK FOR TECHNOLOGISTS AND TECHNICIANS

Although the Institute of Medicine suggests a trend favoring more technologists and expects demand for lower level personnel to be strengthened by shortages among technologists, there is no consensus about what the future holds for technologists as compared with technicians. As the Bureau of Labor Statistics notes:

Employers' preferences vary so much that it is hard to generalize about future prospects for the different levels of clinical laboratory personnel. On the one hand, demand for technologists is likely to be sustained by the complexity of much clinical testing; the need for in-depth knowledge and independent judgment to verify test results and advise physicians; expansion of research laboratory facilities; and technologists' greater versatility. . . . On the other hand, advances in laboratory automation will continue to routinize certain tests, which may be favorable for technicians. . . . Like other areas of health care, the clinical laboratory is undergoing change on a scale that makes it extremely difficult to project future trends. For both technologists and technicians, demand will vary among employment settings, and job prospects will be affected by diverse factors including economic conditions; structure of the clinical laboratory market; strategies by health care providers seeking to enter the market; third-party reimbursement policy and other profit considerations; and changes in laboratory [personnel] licensure and staffing regulations.

Most experts within the profession would agree that extreme caution is warranted in predicting how key questions will affect the outlook for the two practitioner levels.

1. Will the scientist's versatility and productivity offset his or her higher salary as contrasted with the technician?
2. Will technology increase or reduce demand for less educated technicians or more educated scientists?
3. How will laws and regulations on practitioner qualifications affect demand?
4. Will laws change where necessary to expand certain forms of independent practice for clinical laboratory scientists?
5. As technology generates more and more "user-friendly" test kits, will it also generate new career paths to offset any resulting drop in demand for technicians or scientists?

SALARIES OUTLOOK

Results of several recent studies show that salaries and benefits are rising across all categories and levels of practice. In some areas, employers are offering bonuses such as tuition credits; relocation expenses; housing assistance; and one-time, lump-sum payments.

According to a recent survey, the number of laboratory administrators anticipating improved laboratory salaries over the coming five years grew from only thirteen percent in late 1986 to fifty-six percent in late 1988.

These findings mark the beginning of a very strong market for qualified medical technologists for the foreseeable future. They also mark the end of 1984–1985 slow hiring environment resulting both from massive federal cost containment efforts and from related, exaggerated pessimism on the part of many employment forecasts.

In addition, they reflect the industry's sturdy resilience in the face of massive economic changes that transformed even hospital laboratories into lean, profit-oriented business centers. Today, any laboratory that withstood these changes shows at least some degree of shrewd management and good marketing, and probably shows expanded test volumes and enhanced profitability.

Virtually all profession leaders predict rising salaries, citing the personnel shortage, declines in the prospective labor pool, improved institutional profitability, increased demand for services, and to a lesser extent, unionization. (According to the IOM, only twenty percent of medical technologists are unionized.)

First, experts predict that the number of women in the labor force as a whole will increase at more than twice the pace of the number of men, and by 2000, women will constitute half the work force. Second, they predict a decline in the number of college-educated persons in the United States by the year 2000. As a result, the economy as a whole will be more dependent on college-educated women than at any time in the past. Science-based, highly technical fields especially will be less able to offset this pressure through reliance on less well-educated workers and will be more competitive with each other for fewer qualified graduates. That will increase pressures on traditionally female, science-based fields like clinical laboratory science and other allied health professions to make their salaries more attractive. As noted health policy analyst Ewe Reinhardt in "Somber Clouds on the Horizon," *Health Week* 1, no. 10 (December 1987), 23:6, put it:

> Gone are the days when doctors and hospitals could look upon America's bright and motivated women as a source of cheap labor denied economic opportunities elsewhere. To attract this pool of talented workers into health care, we must get used to the notion of paying competitive wages.

As this occurs, such professions will become more attractive to men *and* women.

Even in boom times, salary levels vary from locale to locale, and even from employer to employer according to local supply and demand and underlying economic forces. Therefore, the figures that follow should be taken only as broad indications of salary levels as they were in late 1988. For current, actual figures, contact the personnel office at several hospitals and clinical laboratories in your area.

Two recent surveys showing both rising salaries and salary levels as they stood in late 1988, are summarized in table 1.1. Because the two were conducted using different methods, they should not be read as comparable. All they can do is show approximately what average salaries looked like at that time.

Table 1.1. Reported Average Salary Levels (All Labs) Late 1988.

Staff Level	*Benezra*[1]	*ASCP*[2]
Manager	$34,400	$28,800–38,600
Chief	$28,000	N/A
Supervisor	$24,900	$23,400–32,300
Staff Scientist/Technologist	$20,200	$19,822–27,000
Technician	$15,800	$15,900–21,300
Phlebotomist	N/A	N/A
Supervisor Cytotechnologist	N/A	$23,400–32,600
Staff Cytotechnologist	N/A	$19,800–27,500
Supervisor Histotechnologist	N/A	$22,400–30,100
Staff Histotechnologist	N/A	$16,700–23,000

[1]Nat Benezra. "Lab Salaries: Still Too Low But Rising, Part I," *Medical Laboratory Observer* (January 1989), 22. These figures represent average current starting salaries.
[2]ASCP. "Salary and Vacancy Study of Medical Laboratories," Market Opinion Research for American Society of Clinical Pathologists. Unpublished. Released 11/30/88. These figures represent *median* average salaries at starting and experienced levels.

For staff technologists, according to the ASCP study for 1988, hospitals performing between 100,000 and 500,000 tests a year pay highest median salaries, and large city/suburban hospitals pay higher median salaries than any other employer category surveyed. Salaries for these practitioners are reported to be best in the West, followed in order by the Northeast, the South Central Atlantic; the East North Central and West South Central; and the West North Central. And federal hospitals pay more than nonfederal hospitals. In general, the Benezra report showed similar regional patterns, and also noted that medium-sized hospitals outperformed smaller institutions.

JOB SATISFACTION

Medical technology is an extremely rewarding profession for bright, science-oriented individuals who wish to apply a rich, broad-based body of knowledge to health care. Built on a curriculum analogous to pre-medicine, medical technology integrates several bioscience disciplines as well as physiology, pathology, and, increasingly, computer and management sciences. This makes a baccalaureate degree in this field an excellent springboard for a great many career options.

Though this is changing, historically clinical laboratory professionals have looked to themselves for knowledge of a job well done. Few people within, and fewer outside, the health care system understand their demanding roles in the "control room" of health services delivery. Even the many patients whose lives have been saved by a laboratory professional are likely to be vague about the high-tech laboratory world.

Public awareness of the field is increasing, however. The technological advantages that have made testing for substance abuse a multi-million dollar industry, and the appalling AIDS tragedy, symbolically have brought the laboratory from the depths of the hospital to the public's living room. Today, most people understand the risks to themselves of an inaccurate cocaine test, or the potential for harm if a positive HIV screen is read as negative. Increasingly, thanks to these easily understood examples of medical technology, the public is learning to appreciate the laboratory professional's skill and dedication. As the shortage increases, public awareness will increase even further, through media recruitment efforts and, potentially, increased publicity about possible declines in test quality and reliability resulting from the shortage.

Clinical laboratory science is an exacting, precise profession. It rewards the abilities of the competent practitioner with the knowledge that his or her skill and persistence have saved a life, discovered the organic cause of a rare disorder, cracked a stubborn diagnostic problem, prevented a lethal transfusion, or found the obscure fact that starts the patient on the road to recovery.

Clinical laboratory science brings unique satisfactions. Clinical laboratory scientists are health care investigators who journey to the center of life and see its many mysteries up close. Those who work in large medical center and research laboratories are responsible for millions of dollars worth of state-of-the-art technology and have the opportunity to work with techniques and tools at the forefront of clinical diagnostic research. That is because the increasing applicability of advances in electronics, the microchip, genetics, laser technologies, biosensors, and other fields make the clinical laboratory one of the first centers of deployment for new soft and hard technologies.

Wherever they work, their skills are required in situations ranging from the discovery of a new pregnancy to the fast-paced, life-and-death intensity of the emergency room and operating theater. Medical technologists are among the few health care professionals to experience the challenge of the entire range of human disorders or the joys of the human being's full health potential.

Medical diagnosis and good health care depend on the technologists' knowledge and integrity. Because it is essential to the mission of the attending physician, the surgeon, the nurse, the pharmacist, the physical and respiratory therapist, and other members of the health care team, medical technology can be an extremely demanding field. Much of the technologist's work must be done quickly and all of it must be accurate. Results have to be sped to the attending physician; an operation may be in progress. There is no margin for error because mistakes in the laboratory may mean costly foul-ups in medical care, critical illness, and even death.

Like any other, this profession has aspects that have to be balanced against its many advantages. Within clinical practice, opportunities for advancement are somewhat modest; as with any hierarchy, there are fewer senior than entry-level positions. Also, although the rich diversity in the profession's knowledge base permits numerous career paths, there remain peculiarities resulting from competition with pathologists that can frustrate the qualified medical technologist's advancement within some laboratories.

Stress, too, is an occupational hazard for professionals in clinical practice. Demands for quick results come not only from attending physicians and nurses, but also from managers oriented to the bottom line who often stress that "time is money." Those pressures are worsened by personnel shortages because fewer staff are available to handle the workload.

Image, too, is an issue. Because the public is less aware of this profession than of other health care fields, medical technologists get less credit than they deserve. Most experts believe that the shortage will result in much more publicity, though, and improved public awareness will bring increased personal satisfaction.

Finally, although salaries are rising—at a rate of six percent to twelve percent in some areas in 1988 alone—and although benefits and other incentives are also improving quickly, most practitioners feel that clinical laboratory salaries lag behind those of other health care professions. Reasons often cited include the profession's low public profile; carryover practices permitting entrance into the field via nonbaccalaureate routes; blurred job descriptions; and intraprofessional disagreements about personnel standards and job descriptions that make bargaining with hospital administrators and other employers difficult, if not impossible.

Certainly one factor not unique to medical technology is that the majority of its practitioners are women. According to the Institute of Medicine, in *Allied Health Services: Avoiding Crises,* "compensation for the allied health professions should be understood in the context of women's earnings, because women [predominate in] many allied health fields. In 1986, women earned on average 69.2 cents for every dollar earned by men. Moreover, occupations in which women represent the majority of workers tend to rank lower in terms of earnings than male dominated occupations."

Although almost everywhere, experts agree, starting salaries are reasonably strong, the IOM further claims that "[i]ncreases in earnings over the length of a career are substantially lower in allied health fields than in [selected] other occupations." This is among the serious issues that employers must address for all allied health professions and for nursing as well, in order to attract new recruits and prevent experienced professionals from leaving the field.

FINANCIAL REQUIREMENTS

The cost of a baccalaureate education in clinical laboratory science is similar to that in nursing or occupational therapy. Often, the first two to three preprofessional years are taken in a liberal arts setting in biology or chemistry. In public institutions, tuition may range from $1,000 to $4,000–5,000 per year. In private colleges and universities, tuition is much the same as that for other science majors and may cost up to $10,000 per year.

Tuition for the professional component of laboratory sciences education is variable, and may be the same as during the preprofessional period. Because of the shortage of laboratory personnel, some hospitals may also offer stipends as incentives to students, in the hope that they will remain in that laboratory as employees, following graduation.

A variety of scholarships are available to students, especially once they are in the professional program. Scholarships are provided by the American Society for Medical Technology (ASMT) and its state societies, as well as other organizations. Loans and grants may also be acquired; information can be obtained at the financial aid office of the college or university that one is attending.

CONCLUSION

Clinical laboratory science represents exciting opportunities for individuals interested in science, technology, and helping humankind. Those in the field who enjoy their work state these reasons for high job satisfaction:

- pride in the profession
- sense of accomplishment in work that is well done
- the nature of the work: challenging, interesting
- use of cutting-edge technologies

- use of problem-solving abilities
- team effort and spirit
- interaction with other health providers
- recognition as a care-giver
- sense of being needed
- sense of independence, little supervision needed
- employment opportunities immediately following graduation and thereafter

CHAPTER 2

WORK SITES

OVERVIEW

Medical technologists today are found in many settings—almost everywhere professional health services are provided. Opportunities exist here and abroad and in traditional settings, such as hospitals, and nontraditional settings, such as the Peace Corps.

That wasn't always the case. As we'll discuss further in chapter 7, "Issues for the Profession and the Practitioner," in the early days, the forerunner of today's professional worked exclusively in a hospital-based laboratory as an aide to a physician called a pathologist, a specialist in the branch of medicine concerned with the study of the nature of disease and its physiological causes and consequences. Today, thanks to rapid advances in test technology and demand for laboratory services, laboratories are no longer confined to hospitals, and laboratory professionals fulfill much broader responsibilities.

LABORATORY DISTRIBUTION

Most laboratory tests are performed in one of three facilities: hospital laboratories; laboratories geographically and administratively independent from hospitals; and laboratories in physicians' offices, or clinics.

In 1976, the Laboratory Management Consultation Office at the Centers for Disease Control (Atlanta, Georgia) updated a 1971 survey conducted by the American Society for Medical Technology (ASMT). That survey indicated the laboratory distribution shown in table 2.1.

Table 2.1 Distribution of U.S. Laboratories, 1976.

Type	Number	Percent of Total
Hospital	7,235	53.1
(Federal)	(528)	(3.9)
(State, county, city)	(2,156)	(15.8)
(Nongovernmental)	(4,551)	(33.4)
Private (independent)	3,163	23.2
Group practice	1,731	12.7
Outpatient clinic	461	3.4
Health department	411	3.0
Industrial	89	0.7
Health Maintenance Organization	75	0.6
Other	461	3.4

Courtesy of Karen R. Karni, "Table 1-2, 'Number of U.S. Laboratories Classified by Supporting Agency and Settings, 1971–1976,' " in "An Overview," *Clinical Laboratory Management: A Guide for Clinical Laboratory Scientists* (Boston: Little, Brown and Co., Inc.), p. 7.

Since the 1976 survey was conducted, several developments have occurred that significantly changed the distribution of laboratory tests (i.e., where most tests are performed) and therefore, the distribution of laboratories. One in particular affected the entire health services delivery system. Since other policies with the same general consequences are expected for the foreseeable future, the federal health care cost containment strategy initiated in 1983 is worth a brief digression.

Government-Regulated Laboratories

In its capacity as a major purchaser of health care services for Medicare and Medicaid beneficiaries, the federal government exerts an enormous influence on the health care service delivery marketplace. Medicare alone is estimated to account for about forty percent of a hospital's patient revenues and a huge share of the six billion tests performed each year at an annual cost of between $20 and $25 billion. Therefore, any change in how Medicare pays for the services it purchases on behalf of its Medicare beneficiaries will influence how the providers of those services operate their businesses. That certainly has been the case since 1983.

That year, to try to control runaway health care costs, the federal government adopted a program called Prospective Payment, which in effect put hospitals on an annual allowance. It forced hospitals to keep the bill to the federal government for inpatient Medicare services within the allowed amount, or made them absorb the difference. Overall, the Prospective Payment program gave hospitals the incentive to perform fewer and fewer inpatient tests, and more and more outpatient tests. Other changes later affected outpatient tests, too.

Because of such sweeping regulatory changes, and also because of the peculiar way in which the federal government regulated laboratories until 1989—different federal regulations applied to different laboratories depending on their site—precise numbers for U.S. laboratories are impossible to obtain. Independent labs were generally subjected to more detailed regulation than hospital labs, and the vast majority of physician office labs were entirely unregulated. Since the federal government has the means to count only the labs it regulates, and since laboratories exist in such an array of facilities, it has never been possible to count precisely all the laboratories in all settings.

Nevertheless, experts estimate that the number of laboratories in nonhospital settings has increased significantly, while hospitals—and therefore hospital laboratories—have decreased.

As of 1988, through its role as major purchaser, and in its capacity as preserver of the public good, the U.S. government is estimated to regulate some 12,000 of an estimated total of over 100,000 clinical laboratories.[1]

---

[1]Report 100-899 to accompany H.R. 5150, U.S. House of Representatives, Committee on Energy and Commerce, 100th Congress, 2nd session, pp. 11–12.

Of these 12,000 regulated laboratories, 6,600 are hospital laboratories, and 4,500 are independent, noninterstate commercial laboratories. Nine hundred are in physicians' offices and other settings, and an additional 1,839 are laboratories engaged in interstate commerce that may be either large hospital facilities or independent, commercial facilities but mostly are the latter.[2]

As those figures suggest, until as recently as December 1988, regulations by federal, state, and local governments that impose personnel standards have had considerable influence on where medical technologists work. In general, they work in regulated settings. In addition to the figures just shown for federal laboratory regulation, forty-eight states regulate hospital laboratories, forty-five states regulate independent laboratories, while only sixteen states regulate physician office laboratories, or POLs (1988 data).

Today, experts estimate that sixty percent of all medical technologists work in hospital or medical center laboratories. Hospitals are usually described by their organizational administrative structure (for instance, "not-for-profit," and "for-profit"), their ownership (federal government, military, private, and municipal), and the number of beds they offer for patient care. Most clinical laboratory practitioners work in small hospitals, with fewer than one hundred beds.

For-Profit Laboratories

Other laboratory personnel work in independent (commercial) laboratories. The remainder work in group medical practice laboratories, physician office laboratories, health maintenance organizations (HMOs), blood banks (such as those in Red Cross facilities), public health laboratories and clinics, emergency and other outpatient centers, and research laboratories.

Of all settings, POLs are believed to employ the fewest numbers of laboratory professionals. That is because, until Congress enacted the Clinical Laboratory Improvement Act of 1988, most physician offices

---

[2]The 1,839 figures include both the 519 *CLIA*-exempt labs accredited by CAP and New York state, and the 1,320 *CLIA*-licensed laboratories.

were not federally regulated.[3] Except in those few cases where state law intervened, this has meant that small POLs performing tests exclusively for their own patients have not been required to meet federal or state personnel standards. Therefore, they have been able to employ nurses, and even secretaries and receptionists, to perform their laboratory tests.

LABORATORY SETTINGS

Small Hospitals

Most health care laboratories, such as those in hospitals, are organized into sections by the type of work performed there. In small hospitals, such as those with fewer than one hundred beds, the laboratory may be divided into the following areas:

- chemistry and urinalysis
- hematology and coagulation
- microbiology including bacteriology, parasitology, and mycology
- blood banking and serology (also called immunology)

In a small hospital, all laboratory sections would most likely be in one room, with specific areas delineated for each kind of analysis, such as chemistry or hematology. In the small hospital laboratory, the staff would probably include a medical technologist laboratory administrator who performs procedures, one other baccalaureate technologist, three laboratory technicians, and a part-time secretary. Persons would be expected to perform all tests, work evenings, and take "call."

---

[3]Unless repealed, *CLIA 88* provisions for physician office laboratories, called POLs, will affect only those POLs performing more than 5,000 tests annually, and will commence in 1991. However, the status of federal personnel standards for laboratories of all types is uncertain at this writing. Depending upon the outcome of current debates about personnel standards for laboratory practitioners, regulation of POLs under *CLIA 88* could have little effect on employment trends in that setting, despite the growing volume of tests performed there.

Medium Hospitals

In a medium sized hospital, e.g. one hundred to four hundred beds, the laboratory would most likely be divided into sections discrete from one another. Typical staff size will vary based on the patient clientele and focus of the hospital (see table 2.2). Thus a 150-bed suburban general care hospital may employ only twenty persons in the laboratory, while a smaller pediatrics hospital employs considerably more laboratory personnel.

Large Hospitals

In a large hospital, one would expect many specialty and subspecialty areas. For example, chemistry might include drug analysis, enzymology, endocrinology, electrolytes, a stat (emergency) lab, and urinalysis. Laboratory personnel would vary in number, from eighty to over five hundred, and are likely to work on fixed shifts, either day, evening, or night. Most laboratories pay differentials—hourly bonuses—for evening and night shifts. These shift differentials are also rising as the shortage of personnel deepens.

Independent Laboratories

If one chooses an independent (commercial) laboratory in which to work, one would expect staff specialization, a profit orientation, sophisticated instrumentation, perhaps a production line approach to test performance. Patient contact would be limited, since specimens are obtained elsewhere and brought to the laboratory. Normally, there would be very little weekend or evening work, although more independent laboratories are operating twenty-four hours each day, seven days a week. In such cases, staffing needs are met through rotating or fixed shift assignments.

Table 2.2
Various Laboratory Settings and Numbers/Kinds of Personnel Employed.

Children's Acute Care Hospital
130 beds

28 medical technologists
19 medical laboratory technicians
3 histologic technicians
12 phlebotomists, EKG
___ technicians, others
62 Total

Suburban Hospital
150 beds

13 medical technologists
2 medical laboratory technicians
_3 clerks
18 Total

Independent (Commercial)
Laboratory
19 medical technologists
10 medical laboratory technicians
6 cytotechnologists
12 phlebotomists
12 specimen processors
6 client clerks
5 lab assistants
11 couriers (drivers)
81 Total

HMO (including 8 small group
practice clinics)
6 medical technologists
23 medical laboratory technicians
_8 phlebotomists/receptionists
37 Total

University Hospital (includes teaching and research mission)
580 beds

358 medical technologists
25 medical laboratory technicians
3 cytotechnologists
4 histologic technicians
9 scientists (Ph.D. level)
14 phlebotomists
11 nurses
2 autopsy technicians
_3 EKG technicians
429 Total

RESEARCH

Research—both basic and applied—is an intriguing area of work, and chosen by a number of laboratorians. Basic research may involve, for

Table 2.2 (*continued*)

Suburban Hospital
400 beds
32 technologists
6 medical laboratory technicians
2 cytotechnologists
5 histologic technicians
7 phlebotomists
3 specimen handlers
17 clerks
72 Total

County Acute Care Hospital
515 beds
79 technologists
16 laboratory technicians
2 cytotechnologists
6 histologic technicians
47 "others" including health
care specialists, phlebotomists,
___ media preparers, computer clerks
150 Total

Ambulatory Care Clinic
(285 physicians, 15 clinic sites)
26 medical technologists
63 medical laboratory technicians
6 lab aids
5 phlebotomists
4 client service representatives
110 Total

Regional Blood Bank

41 medical technologists
13 medical laboratory technicians
5 clerks
59 Total

example, the DNA sequencing of a red cell membrane protein. Applied research may be concerned with trying to obtain the best chemotherapy regimen to use in treating leukemia, or in understanding the immunologic changes that occur with aging. Research provides in-depth expertise in a small area of scientific inquiry; it also provides the opportunity to perform tests, analyze the data, and try to determine the significance of those data. Research may involve only a small amount of patient contact, and interaction with others is usually less frequent than in a hospital setting.

PUBLIC HEALTH

Another area in which laboratory professionals work is in public health. Here, the identification of organisms causing outbreaks of infectious and communicable diseases are made. A variety of immunologic tests are also performed to determine one's prior exposure to mumps, measles, or other diseases. Laboratory analyses for water purity, food safety, and environmental hazards are also performed.

BLOOD BANKS

Blood banks employ a fair number of laboratory personnel. In these organizations, such as those of the American Red Cross, blood is drawn, typed, checked for any unexpected antibodies, as well as for infectious agents such as the hepatitis or AIDS virus, or syphilis spirochete. There is a strong spirit within blood banks, as physicians, nurses, and laboratorians work together to provide safe blood for the community.

INDUSTRY

Industry is attractive to laboratorians who have an entrepreneurial spirit. Here one can work in research and development (R & D), developing new tests or instrumentation, as a technical specialist assisting users who are having problems (e.g. in troubleshooting), or in sales.

SMALL HEALTH CARE FACILITIES

If one works in a clinic, health maintenance organization, or physician office laboratory, the kind and volume of testing depends on the size of the laboratory. The central laboratory of a large HMO, for example, might be very similar to that of a large hospital. However, the lab in a three-physician practice may offer only ten of fifteen tests. In the latter case, only twenty to forty analyses might be performed each day.

Organization of Laboratories

Laboratories are typically organized in a familiar chain-of-command model. At the top are directors and administrators; in the middle are technical supervisory staff; and on the front line, performing the actual tests, are the staff technologists and technicians and phlebotomists.

Of course there are variations on this basic structure. In the hospital, for instance, the laboratory's organization depends on the hospital's size, the types of patients it serves (e.g., pediatric, psychiatric, or acute care), and its objectives. Most hospital laboratories are headed by a director. In many, that individual is a physician specializing in pathology, although in smaller hospitals, qualified nonphysicians, including clinical laboratory scientists and other personnel, assume administrative responsibility and work with a consulting pathologist who assumes medical responsibility. In another model, a physician (usually a pathologist) holds the title "medical director," and a clinical laboratory scientist holds the title "administrative director." Under this arrangement, the physician is responsible for medical interpretive and consultative functions and for anatomical pathology tests while the administrative director colleague manages and administers the facility. In the independent laboratory sector, it is quite common for nonphysician professionals to own, direct, and operate full-service laboratories. (See table 2.3 for an example of an organizational chart for a medium to large hospital laboratory.)

According to standards proposed by the American Society for Medical Technology, under the shared medical/administrative director model, responsibilities are divided to draw most fully on each professional's expertise. In this model, the physician director is in charge of physician-patient services and has the following responsibilities as well:

1. To assist in the establishment of policies and test protocols.
2. To provide consultation services related to requests for tests and interpretation of laboratory data to medical and dental staff.
3. To represent the clinical laboratory staff at medical and dental conferences.
4. To teach in primary and continuing education programs for medical and dental staff and laboratory staff.
5. To provide consultation and interpretation on surgical and autopsy tissues, cytologic specimens, bone marrows, and other specimens.

The laboratory administrator, who, like the medical director, also reports to a senior member of the hospital administration, has day-to-day responsibility for laboratory operations:

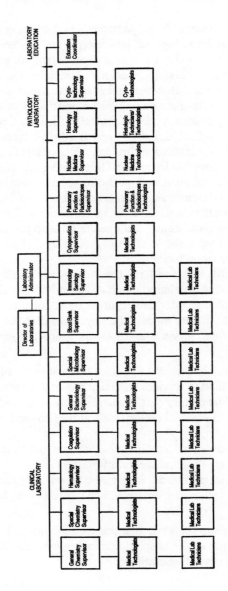

Table 2.3   Clinical Laboratory/Pathology Laboratory Organization Chart for a Medium to Large Hospital

1. To establish all laboratory procedures and quality control practices including responsibility for the preparation and maintenance of an up-to-date procedural manual for each category of services offered by the clinical laboratory.
2. To ensure the availability of technical supervision as required; to employ qualified personnel who will maintain the work flow and quality control standards of the laboratory.
3. To ensure the proper performance of all procedures.
4. To perform the budgetary functions of the laboratory.
5. To provide for orientation and training of new personnel, continuing education of technical and supervisory staff, and assignment of duties to personnel commensurate with their qualifications.
6. To be available for consultation.

The technical supervisor in each of the departments of the laboratory assumes the following responsibilities:

1. To implement quality control practices to ensure the accuracy and validity of test results and procedures.
2. To prepare daily work schedules to provide adequate coverage and effective utilization of personnel.
3. To maintain levels of supplies and reagents commensurate with work load.
4. To ensure that policies, procedures, and safety practices are followed by employees.
5. To provide technical instructions and training of personnel in techniques, instrumentation, and organization of work.
6. To assist the laboratory administrator in preparation of a budget, recommending personnel, supplies, and equipment needs.
7. To maintain a current procedural manual, reviewing and revising as needed, at least once a year.
8. To maintain equipment and instruments in good operating condition, recognizing any malfunctions and taking corrective actions.
9. To provide direct supervision of personnel.

10. To recommend to the laboratory administrator the selection, transfer, discipline, and discharge of personnel.

Technical personnel include technologists (clinical laboratory scientists) and technicians. An abbreviated description of duties and responsibilities of the technologist includes the following:

1. To perform tests that require the exercise of independent judgment and responsibility, with minimal supervision by the director or supervisor.
2. To perform procedures, report results, and maintain equipment, records, and other quality control requirements related to test performance.
3. To provide personal and direct supervision for technologist trainees, technicians, technical trainees, and other supportive technical personnel employed by the laboratory.

Duties and responsibilities for the laboratory technician are:

1. To perform those procedures that require limited exercise of independent judgment.
2. To execute procedures under the supervision of a technologist, supervisor, or director.
3. To follow instructions detailed in the procedural manual for those designated duties; to perform those procedures for which they are qualified by education, training, and experience.

ADVANTAGES AND DISADVANTAGES OF WORKING IN VARIOUS LABORATORY SETTINGS

Hospital and independent laboratories now tend to be more alike than different. That is, they tend to perform services requiring similar practitioner expertise using the same types of instruments. While differences do still exist, today Prospective Payment, discussed earlier, has blurred many traditional lines between the two. This it has done by requiring all laboratory types to compete effectively with each other, or cease to exist.

These days, all kinds of services delivery variations exist. Some independent laboratories perform rare procedures on referral from physicians and hospital labs—procedures that hospitals and large group practices find too costly to offer. Other independent laboratories provide all types of tests. On the other hand, some hospitals refer most of their tests to commercial facilities, and keep only an emergency laboratory operation generally staffed round the clock but equipped to provide quite a limited range of tests. At the same time, other hospital laboratories have entered the testing market quite aggressively. They not only do almost all their own tests; they also serve as referral laboratories for other hospitals and act almost like independent laboratories. Test volume can vary from a few hundred tests a year (in a very small POL) to millions of procedures (in large hospital and independent facilities).

Although rapid specimen transit (by air or road courier) and computer technologies have made regional laboratories possible, not all testing can be done long-distance. For that reason, the type of testing a given facility offers depends significantly on the nature of the services provided and the competition nearby. An important factor for hospital laboratories is the patient case-load, and whether the facility is a large, teaching hospital. A facility that serves predominantly cancer patients (an oncology hospital), or a psychiatric hospital would offer a menu of tests significantly different from each other or from a multi-purpose, acute-care hospital. Similarly, a teaching hospital can be expected to offer a wider range of tests—including rare procedures—than a non-teaching hospital.

According to one expert, James M. Maratea, in "Viewpoint: Two Worlds: Independent and Hospital Labs," *Medical Laboratory Observer* (January 1989), p. 16, independent and hospital laboratories differ mainly in the prevailing focus of each. That is, hospital laboratories (like other hospital departments) exist first and foremost to serve the needs of the inpatient, while independent laboratories exist to make a profit.

According to many professionals, there is no such situation as a laboratory that offers all employment advantages. As in every field, there are trade-offs to be made. While the personnel shortage may force laboratories to undergo changes to make themselves optimally attractive to laboratory staff, there are built-in limits to some changes. And while exceptions do exist and no laboratory matches all the stereotypical qualities, in general, to date each type of facility has certain characteristics, shown in table 2.4.

Physician office laboratories and group practice laboratories span a wide range of characteristics. Some physician office laboratories offer only six or eight of the most common tests, are housed in a space the size of an apartment kitchen, and are staffed by one individual—characteristically *not* a laboratory professional. At the other end of the continuum, large group practice laboratories can rival any hospital facility in test variety, the sophistication of the equipment, and the size and diversity of the staff.

Table 2.4 Work Characteristics of Various Laboratory Settings.

A. Small Hospital Laboratory
   Rotation through lab sections, making one a strong generalist; much patient contact; limited test menu; smaller work force; mandatory shift rotation and "taking call"; very strong patient care orientation; much interaction with other health care staff (optimizing a team spirit).

B. Teaching Hospital Laboratory
   Staff specialization; less patient contact; larger test menu; larger work force; more new technology and instrumentation; fixed shift assignments; moderate patient care orientation; some interaction with other health care staff.

C. Independent (Commercial) Laboratory
   Staff specialization; no patient contact; profit-loss orientation (which may include bonuses); production line orientation; good advancement opportunities; very little contact with other health care professionals.

D. Research Laboratory
   Independent work; limited patient contact; opportunities to develop procedures and make decisions; flexible hours; development of in-depth knowledge of a specific area of inquiry; repetitive work; position may be dependent on grant money.

LABORATORY SAFETY

Clinical laboratory professionals are meticulously educated in the safe management and handling of toxic and infectious substances since this is an integral part of the work they do. Therefore, extremely reliable, safe procedures are continually being improved upon and introduced into practice. With the advent of Human Immunodeficiency Virus, these procedures and precautions have been even more intensified, and the universal precautions mandated by the Occupational Safety and Health Administration (OSHA) have drastically minimized any risk of accidental exposure.

Over time, plastics and disposables have widely replaced glass instruments, and chemical burns are extremely rare in healthcare laboratories because many reagents in use today are premixed and prepackaged.

Table 2.4 (*continued*)

E. Public Health Laboratory
Work heavily microbiology and immunology oriented; very little patient contact; may involve routine testing; no weekend work; little interaction with other health professionals.

F. Blood Bank
Strong commitment (organizational and individual) to providing safe blood and blood products for transfusion; specialized work; little direct patient contact; some donor contact; considerable interaction with other health professionals, especially physicians and nurses.

G. Industry (Example: development of new lab tests or instrumentation)
Emphasis on scientific entrepreneurship and profit-making; may require knowledge of government regulations; work may be repetitive; no patient contact; limited interaction with other health professionals; good opportunities for advancement.

H. Clinic/HMO/Physician Office Laboratory (having a small practice)
Very limited test menu (six to twenty tests); diverse work, for example, may include X-ray or record keeping; much patient contact; usually does not include shift or weekend work; strong interaction with clinic/HMO/ physician staff.

Unpleasant odors are not characteristic, thanks to changes in clinical laboratory practice itself, and to biosafety shields, cabinets, and ventilators. Today's clinical laboratory is likely to have a clean, astringent scent, if any at all.

SUMMARY

Opportunities in clinical laboratory practice exist in quite an array of settings, traditional and nontraditional. Depending upon one's interest and qualifications, there are opportunities for technical, supervisory, and management roles, as well as for a host of roles outside the laboratory itself. As today's health care industry continues to change in response to new technologies, added pressures to control health care costs, and new discoveries in science and medicine and clinical laboratory science itself, qualified clinical laboratory practitioners can look forward to an array of options within and outside the conventional laboratory setting.

CHAPTER 3

OVERVIEW OF LABORATORY PERSONNEL

The persons who work in clinical laboratories are as varied as the laboratory settings themselves. While hospitals employ the greatest percentage of laboratory personnel (at least sixty percent), the greatest number of all laboratory technicians are those whom we call "medical technologists" or "clinical laboratory scientists."

It is estimated that the number of laboratory personnel in the United States is at least 250,000, not including those in physician office laboratories and small clinics. How are they distributed, both by number and category? Table 3.1 depicts this information as follows:

Table 3.1 Classification and Numbers of Laboratory Personnel

	Numbers	% of Total
Pathologists (physicians)	13,000	5
Medical technologists	160,000	64
Cytotechnologists	7,000	3
Medical laboratory technicians	30,000	12
Others	40,000	16
	250,000	100

It can be seen that baccalaureate-level medical technologists comprise almost two-thirds of the staffs of clinical laboratories. The next largest category, "other," is very diverse and encompasses those doctorally prepared scientists (such as microbiologists, clinical chemists, and others educated at the Ph.D. level) as well as persons trained on the job.

In order to define the major players and their jobs in clinical laboratories, the following summary descriptions are provided. These summaries are taken in part from the *Allied Health Education Directory*, 1989, Division of Allied Health Education and Accreditation, American Medical Association, 535 North Dearborn Street, Chicago, IL 60610. Review also table 3.2 to gain an overview of the routes to various laboratory careers.

PATHOLOGIST

Job Description

Seventy-five percent of laboratory directors in the United States are pathologists, physicians with advanced training in the study of the nature, structure, and functional changes produced by diseases. There are two branches of pathology: anatomic pathology (AP) and clinical pathology (CP). Anatomic pathologists are those physican specialists who examine tissues from biopsies, surgeries, and autopsies both macroscopically (by eye) and microsopically. They determine whether the tissues are normal, infected, malignant, inflammatory, necrotic, or with other cellular changes. Pathologists may advise other physicians whether and how to treat those patients whose tissues they have examined.

The other branch of pathology is clinical pathology, sometimes called laboratory medicine. Clinical pathologists are responsible for directing the clinical laboratory or its sections, and providing consultation to other physicians regarding test selection, interpretation of results, and diseases associated with various laboratory values. Clinical pathologists head research and development (R & D) efforts concerning new tests, methodologies and instrumentation; they also teach residents, fellows, and other students. Salaries of pathologists vary. When in a residency program, their income is about $22,000 per year, but once in practice, salaries are usually in excess of $100,000 per year.

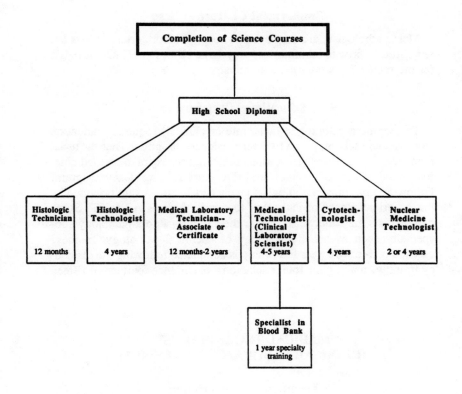

Table 3.2   The Usual Pathways to Laboratory Careers

Employment Characteristics

Most pathologists are employed in hospital laboratories. Others are employed in private laboratories, very large clinics or HMOs, forensic (crime-related) laboratories, and industry.

Educational Programs

To become a pathologist (anatomic or clinical) requires graduation from medical school, plus a five-year residency program. Thus the usual number of years of schooling totals thirteen; four years in premedicine, four years of medical school, and five years in a residency program. Following this, most pathologists take a certification exam provided by the American Board of Pathology to certify them as AP or CP. Some pathologists may choose to further their inquiry into a pathology subspecialty such as hematopathology or chemical pathology. In these cases, a one- or two-year fellowship is completed following the residency training, making the total educational experience fourteen or fifteen years.

MEDICAL TECHNOLOGIST
(CLINICAL LABORATORY SCIENTIST)

Occupational Description

Laboratory test results play a crucial role in the detection, diagnosis, and treatment of many diseases. Medical technologists perform these tests in association with physicians and scientists in clinical chemistry, microbiology, and the other biological sciences. Medical technologists provide data on blood, tissues, and fluids in the human body by using simple procedures as well as those requiring sophisticated instruments and complicated methodologies.

Job Description

Medical technologists perform complex analyses, and use fine line discrimination in determining the correctness of results. They are able to recognize the interdependency of tests and have knowledge of physiological conditions affecting test results in order to confirm such results. In health care settings, they develop data that are used by physicians in determining the presence, extent, and, as far as possible, the cause of disease.

Medical technologists assume responsibility for, and are held accountable for, accurate results. They establish and monitor quality control programs and design or modify procedures as necessary. Tests and procedures are performed or supervised by medical technologists in the clinical laboratory center in the major areas of hematology, coagulation, microbiology, immunohematology, immunology, clinical chemistry, and urinalysis.

Subspecialty areas in which medical technologists work include cytogenetics, fertility testing, flow cytometry, bone and skin banks, forensic laboratories, infection control laboratories, platelet and neutrophil studies laboratories, tissue typing, and others.

Employment Characteristics

The majority of clinical laboratory scientists are employed in hospital laboratories. The remainder are employed in HMOs; private laboratories and clinics; by the armed forces; by city, state, and federal health agencies; in industrial medical laboratories; in pharmaceutical houses; in numerous public and private research programs; and as faculty of programs preparing medical laboratory personnel. Salaries vary depending on the employer and geographic location. According to a 1989 survey of program directors, salaries of entry-level medical technologists averaged $22,000.

The job market for medical technologists is excellent. There were over 12,000 vacancies for staff technologists alone in 1989. Another 6,000 vacancies existed for supervisors and administrators.

Educational Programs

Most medical technologists are graduates of baccalaureate programs, which include a professional component of one to two years. In colleges and universities which offer the preprofessional curriculum, but are not themselves accredited in medical technology, students usually complete three years of school in a curriculum that is close to that of a premedical student. Prerequisite courses include general chemistry, general biology, organic and/or biochemistry, mathematics, microbiology, immunology, and perhaps computer science. Optional courses may include physics and statistics. Students then spend one year in an accredited "school" of medical technology, usually located in a hospital. Here, instruction and laboratory experiences are provided in hematology, chemistry, microbiology, immunohematology, and immunology.

In California, the majority of medical technology programs are of the 4 + 1 model: 4 years in college followed by a 1-year clinical internship.

In colleges and universities, which are themselves accredited in clinical laboratory science or medical technology, students usually spend two years in a preprofessional program and two years in a professional program. The first two years are spent in completing prerequisites in general chemistry, general biology, organic chemistry, mathematics, and microbiology, again, in a curriculum resembling that of a premedical student. At the third year, students complete course work in computer science, immunology, anatomy, and physiology and begin taking preclinical (introductory) laboratory courses in clinical chemistry, hematology, microbiology, and immunohematology. These introductory courses are usually conducted in student laboratories. Further courses in pathophysiology, management, and education are provided, and in the final (fourth) year the actual hospital experience is shortened to twenty to thirty-five weeks. In this 2 + 2 model, students start their laboratory work in year three, and the preprofessional and professional course work are integrated. This type of program is usually found in academic health science centers and medical schools.

Upon meeting specified qualifications and passing an examination, these professionals may be certified by one or more voluntary certifying agencies as generalists. Individuals are usually certified by the National Certification Agency for Medical Laboratory Personnel (NCA) or the Board of Registry of the American Society of Clinical Pathologists (ASCP).

CYTOTECHNOLOGIST

Occupational Description

Cytology is the study of the structure and the function of cells. Cytotechnologists are trained medical laboratory technologists who work with pathologists to detect changes in body cells which may be important in the early diagnosis of cancer. This is done primarily with the microscope used to screen slide preparations of body cells for abnormalities in structure, indicating either benign or malignant conditions.

Job Description

Using special techniques, cytotechnologists prepare cellular samples for study under the microscope and assist in the diagnosis of disease by the examination of the samples. Cell specimens may be obtained from various body sites, such as the female reproductive tract (Pap smears), the oral cavity, the lung, or any body cavity shedding cells. Examination is made of abdominal fluids, thoracic fluids, central nervous system fluids, urine, sputum, and cells obtained by brushing the surfaces of various organs. Using the findings of cytotechnologists, the physician is then able in many instances to diagnose cancer long before it can be detected by other methods. Cytologic techniques are also used to detect diseases involving hormonal abnormalities and other pathological disease processes. In recent years fine needles have been used to aspirate lesions, often deeply seated in the body, thus greatly enhancing the ability to diagnose tumors located in inaccessible sites.

Employment Characteristics

Most cytotechnologists work in hospitals or in private laboratories, while others prefer to work on research projects or to teach. Employment opportunities are excellent, as the demand for trained cytotechnologists is high and is projected to remain high.

According to information supplied in a 1989 survey of program directors, entry-level salaries of cytotechnologists averaged $22,000 per year.

Educational Programs

The length of the cytotechnology program depends significantly on its organizational structure. In general, after completion of three years of prerequisite course work, at least one calendar year of structured professional instruction in cytotechnology is necessary to establish entry-level competencies.

Applicants should be well grounded in the biological sciences and in basic chemistry. This usually entails successful completion of at least twenty semester hours in the biological sciences, chemistry courses equaling or exceeding eight semester hours, and some mathematics.

The curriculum includes the historical background of cytology, cytology as applied in clinical medicine, cytology in the screening of exfoliate tumor cells, and areas of anatomy, histology, embryology, cytochemistry, cytophysiology, endocrinology, and inflammatory diseases.

Like medical technology, some schools provide 2 + 2 curricula in cytotechnology, once again providing preclinical cytology courses in year three, and offering in-depth instruction in cell identification, fine needle biopsy examination, and the like.

MEDICAL (CLINICAL) LABORATORY TECHNICIAN

Occupational Description

Medical laboratory technicians (associate or certificate) perform many routine procedures in the clinical laboratory under the direction of a qualified physician and/or medical technologist.

Job Description

Medical laboratory technicians perform routine, uncomplicated procedures in the areas of hematology, serology, blood banking, urinalysis, microbiology, and clinical chemistry. These procedures involve the use of common laboratory instruments in processes where discrimination is clear, errors are few and easily corrected, and results of the procedures can be confirmed with a reference test or source within the working area. The technician has knowledge of specific techniques and instruments and is able to recognize factors that directly affect procedures and results. The technician also monitors quality control programs which have predetermined parameters.

Employment Opportunities

Some medical laboratory technicians (MLTs), also called CLTs, work in hospital laboratories, averaging a forty-hour week; many more technicians work in HMOs, clinics, and physician office laboratories.

According to a 1989 survey, entry-level salaries of certificate-level medical laboratory personnel averaged $16,000–$17,000.

Educational Programs

Medical laboratory technicians have two routes to choose in completing an MLT program. The first is the MLT certificate (MLT-C) program, which is usually twelve to fifteen months in length, and often located at a vocational or technical institute or college. Here, the curriculum includes areas of medical ethics and conduct, medical terminology, basic laboratory solutions and media, basic elements of quality control, blood collecting techniques, basic microbiology, hematology, serology, and immunohematology. A clinical practicum in a hospital or clinic laboratory concludes the MLT-C program.

The second route to becoming a medical laboratory technician involves completion of an associate degree (MLT-AD) usually at a junior or community college. The period of education is usually two academic years. Courses are taught on campus and in affiliated hospital(s). The teaching laboratory on campus focuses on general knowledge and basic skills, understanding principles, and mastering procedures of laboratory testing. The clinical (hospital) courses include application of basic principles commonly used in the diagnostic laboratory. Technical instruction includes procedures in hematology, serology, chemistry, microbiology, and immunohematology.

If one is planning to become a laboratory technician first and then take additional course work to become a medical technologist, we recommend that the associate level route be chosen. It may be difficult to transfer credits from a vocational or technical school to a college or university. Transfer of credits from a community or junior college can more easily be accomplished.

The medical laboratory technician title may also be designated for those who have graduated as medical laboratory specialists in the armed forces (see chapter 5).

OTHER LABORATORY PERSONNEL

Specialist in Blood Bank Technology

JOB DESCRIPTION:

Specialists in blood bank technology (SBB) demonstrate a superior level of technical proficiency and problem-solving ability in such areas as: 1) testing for blood group antigens, compatibility, and antibody identification; 2) investigating abnormalities such as hemolytic disease of the newborn, hemolytic anemias, and adverse responses to transfusion; 3) supporting physicians in transfusion therapy, including patients with coagulopathies or candidates for homologous organ transplant; 4) blood collection and processing, including selecting donors, drawing and typing blood, and performing pretransfusion tests to ensure the safety of the patient. Supervision, management, and/or teaching comprise a considerable part of the responsibilities of the specialist in blood bank technology.

EMPLOYMENT CHARACTERISTICS:

Specialists in blood banking work in many types of facilities, including community blood centers, private hospital blood banks, university affiliated blood banks, transfusion services, and independent laboratories; they may also be a part of a university faculty. Qualified specialists may advance to supervisory or administrative positions, or move into teaching or research activities.

According to information supplied in a 1989 survey of program directors, entry-level salaries of specialists in blood bank technology averaged $25,000 per year.

EDUCATIONAL PROGRAMS:

The minimum length of the SBB educational program must be twelve consecutive months. Applicants must hold a certificate in medical technology and possess a baccalaureate degree from a regionally accredited college or university. If applicants are not certified in medical technology, they must possess a baccalaureate degree from a regionally accredited college or university with a major in any of the biological or physical sciences.

Each SBB educational program defines its own criteria for measurement of student achievement; the sequence of instruction is at the discretion of the medical director and program director. The educational design and environment are conducive to the development of competence in all technical areas of the modern blood bank and transfusion services.

Nuclear Medical Technologist

OCCUPATIONAL DESCRIPTION:

Nuclear medicine is the medical specialty that utilizes the nuclear properties of radioactive and stable nuclides to make diagnostic evaluations of the anatomic or physiologic conditions of the body and to provide therapy with unsealed radioactive sources.

JOB DESCRIPTION:

Nuclear medicine technologists (NMT) apply their knowledge of radiation physics and safety regulations to limit radiation exposure; prepare and administer radiopharmaceuticals; use radiation detection devices and other kinds of laboratory equipment that measure the quantity and distribution of radionuclides deposited in the patient or in a patient specimen. They perform in vivo and in vitro diagnostic procedures, utilize quality control techniques as part of a quality assurance program covering all procedures and products in the laboratory, and participate in research activities.

Administrative functions may include supervising other nuclear medicine technologists, students, laboratory assistants, and other personnel; procuring supplies and equipment; documenting laboratory operations; participating in departmental inspections conducted by various licensing, regulatory, and accrediting agencies; and scheduling patient examinations.

EMPLOYMENT CHARACTERISTICS:

The employment outlook in nuclear medicine technology is very bright. Opportunities may be found both in major medical centers and in smaller hospitals. Opportunities are also available for obtaining positions in clinical research, education, and administration.

According to a recent survey of program directors, salaries of entry-level nuclear medicine technologists averaged $21,000 per year.

EDUCATIONAL PROGRAMS:

The technical portion of the nuclear medicine program is one year in length. Institutions offering accredited programs may provide an integrated educational sequence leading to an associate or baccalaureate degree over a period of two or four years.

The curriculum includes patient care, nuclear physics, instrumentation and statistics, health physics, biochemistry, immunology, radiopharmacology, administration, radiation biology, clinical nuclear medicine, radionuclide therapy, and introduction to computer application.

Histology Technician/Technologist

OCCUPATIONAL DESCRIPTION:

The main responsibility of the histologic technician/technologist in the clinical laboratory is preparing sections of body tissue for examination by a pathologist. This includes tissue specimens of human and animal origin for diagnostic, research, or teaching purposes.

JOB DESCRIPTION:

Histotechnicians process sections of body tissue by fixation, dehydration, embedding, sectioning, decalcification, microincineration, mounting, and routine and special staining. Histotechnologists perform all the functions of the histotechnician as well as the more complex procedures for processing tissues. They identify tissue structures, cell components, and their staining characteristics, and relate them to physiological functions; implement and test new techniques and procedures; make judgments concerning the results of quality control measures; and institute proper procedures to maintain accuracy and precision. Histotechnologists apply the principles of management and supervision when they function as section supervisors and educational methodology when they teach students.

EMPLOYMENT CHARACTERISTICS:

Most histologic technicians/technologists work in hospital laboratories, averaging a forty-hour week.

According to a 1988 survey entry-level salaries averaged $17,000 for histologic technicians and $22,000 for histologic technologists.

EDUCATIONAL PROGRAM:

Twelve months for histotechnicians, unless the curriculum is an integral part of a college program. For the histotechnologist, a baccalaureate degree program of four years.

CURRICULUM:

The curriculum includes both didactic instruction and practical demonstration in the areas of medical ethics, medical terminology, chemistry, laboratory mathematics, anatomy, histology, histochemistry, quality control, instrumentation, microscopy, processing techniques, preparation of museum specimens, and record and administration procedures.

It has been recommended that the curriculum be an integral part of a junior or community college program culminating in an associate degree, and that the course of study include chemistry, biology, and mathematics. The baccalaureate level program includes course work designed to prepare supervisors and teachers with advanced capabilities.

Phlebotomist

Phlebotomists are those individuals who draw blood from patients for the purposes of analysis. Most blood is obtained by venipuncture, although capillary blood from fingers or babies' heels may be used. In the past many phlebotomists were trained on the job (OJT); now, short courses of six to twenty weeks are provided in hospitals, community and junior colleges, or technical and vocational schools.

Most phlebotomists work in hospitals, but others work in large clinics and HMOs. Phlebotomists are the laboratory personnel who convey to patients the image of the laboratory; therefore it is important that they be highly professional in appearance and manner. Average entry-level salary is approximately $14,000 per year.

A high school diploma or equivalent is usually required. Course work or training includes basic anatomy and physiology (the circulatory system and blood); medical terminology; specimen collection; anticoagulants; patient preparation; techniques; equipment; specimen processing and handling (specimen types, labeling, transport, storage); safety; quality control; infection control; interpersonal relations; and professional ethics.

Other Specialists

In addition to the previously mentioned laboratory personnel, there are other scientists and specialists who work in laboratories. These include doctorally prepared clinical chemists, microbiologists, immunologists, and pathobiologists (Ph.D. level); master's-level personnel in these areas; and other specialists. Such individuals are responsible for administering a laboratory section, performing research, and teaching. They may be medical technologists with advanced degrees, or they may have biology, chemistry, or microbiology backgrounds. They usually are employed in large hospitals, medical centers, and universities. Entry-level salaries vary by degree and experience, but usually begin at $28,000 to $30,000 per year.

Others employed in laboratories include specialists who have advanced by way of additional course work and experience. This group includes specialists in hematology, coagulation, chemistry, microbiology, immunology, or cytogentics. (The latter are those specialists who study the structure and abnormalities of chromosomes, such as Trisomy 21 of Down's syndrome.)

Yet others, whose educational preparation is significantly different from cyto- and histotechnologists, are histocompatibility technologists employed in organ donor centers and transplantation.

PRACTITIONER ATTRIBUTES

Though there are numerous career paths in clinical laboratory science, the core career is clinical laboratory practice. With certain exceptions (generally made explicit in the text), the personal qualifications are similar for technologist and technician practitioners. Additional aptitudes and abilities may be required of management, and fewer educational and other requirements apply to laboratory technicians.

Intellectual Requirements

This science-based, investigative profession requires considerable intelligence and sound problem-solving abilities. Interest and aptitude in science, particularly biology, is essential, and competence in mathematics is necessary. Some compare the technologist's curriculum to the premedicine curriculum, noting that a clinical laboratory science major requires courses in anatomy, physiology, biological science, physics, biochemistry, microbiology, and medical technology.

For supervisors, managers, and directors, requirements are even more stringent. Escalating pressures for cost containment and productivity, and increased computerization, have added computer science, human and fiscal management, and even marketing to the preferred knowledge base. And as competition and technology extend the laboratory's reach beyond the hospital to diverse, ambulatory care settings, good communications and interactive skills are in demand.

Emotional Requirements

Clinical laboratory scientists perform volumes of exacting, precision work under considerable pressure; life-and-death situations often join productivity demands to escalate the pressures under which they perform. They must have a strong desire to help others. The ability to work carefully and quickly under pressure is necessary. These practitioners must also have an extremely high level of integrity and personal responsibility; patients' lives depend on their commitment to provide the highest quality of service. These practitioners must also be emotionally stable, patient, and able to follow detailed written and oral instructions.

Traditionally, except for the phlebotomist, medical technologists had perhaps a greater affinity for scientific, research-, and detail-oriented tasks than for human interaction. While the former aptitudes are still desirable, the professional in the year 2000 is also likely to need solid interpersonal abilities and good communications skills. Phlebotomists may encounter unusual situations since they draw blood specimens directly from patients. They must be, and generally are trained to be, diplomats. They can encounter extreme pressure and even verbal abuse when sick patients resent the inevitable discomforts of illness and are reluctant to express their frustrations to physicians or nurses. These situations can also pertain in laboratories in physicians' offices, where laboratory practitioners have more patient contact. And it is important to note that patients are not always difficult. They can also make for some of the practitioner's most deeply satisfying moments.

Physical Requirements

These professionals often rely on eyesight to assist in specimen examinations. Good physical health and manual dexterity are important characteristics. Standing and walking may be required.

SUMMARY

Clinical laboratories employ a wide variety of personnel, ranging in background from doctorally prepared scientists to on-the-job trained phlebotomists. The largest group employed are medical technologists (clinical laboratory scientists) who comprise about two-thirds of all persons found in laboratories. Nevertheless, the variety of personnel, their backgrounds and qualifications, contribute to the uniqueness of those found working in clinical laboratories.

CHAPTER 4

OPPORTUNITIES WITHIN LABORATORY SCIENCE

Chapters 2 and 3 described the work sites and job descriptions of various laboratory personnel who traditionally have worked in hospital settings. However, once a person has acquired a baccalaureate degree, considered the foundation of laboratory science, he/she has myriad job opportunities not only in health care settings, but elsewhere as well.

EXTENDED CAREER PATHS

The chart, "Extended Career Paths," shows actual positions taken by graduates of the University of Minnesota Bachelor of Science program in medical technology. This chart depicts jobs inside and outside of health; it is arranged by the following groupings:

- Health care or government agencies
- Hospitals and medical centers
- Health care administration
- Management information systems
- Health maintenance organizations
- Consultantships
- Reference/commercial laboratories
- Veterinary medicine
- Working abroad
- Humanitarian work

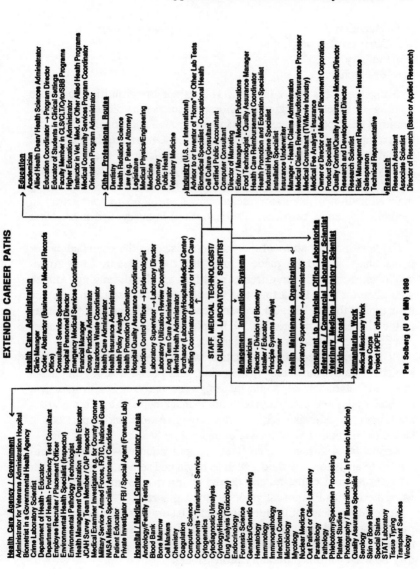

- Education
- Other professions
- Industry
- Research

Altogether, this chart includes 130 career opportunities for those holding a bachelor's degree in laboratory science/medical technology. Some of these positions can be assumed through additional experience, for example, becoming a section supervisor. Others require additional formal education, such as in becoming a physician or academician (a faculty member in a college or university). Nevertheless, the chart includes examples of what medical technologists have become, using their education in laboratory science as a springboard for careers in medicine, science, research, administration, industry, and many other areas.

Explanations for some of the positions listed in the extended career paths chart should be made. Under the title "Health Care Agency/Government," fifteen different positions are listed, ranging from an administrator for a Department of Veterans Affairs hospital to a private investigator for the FBI. The government employs laboratory personnel in the clinical laboratories of VA hospitals and also as administrators and educators within its many agencies.

"Biometrists" are those scientists who analyze mathematical and statistical data from biology, medicine, and public health. Emphases include biostatistics, experimental design and analysis, health statistics, clinical trials, and computerized data management. Often, biometrists are laboratory scientists with additional course work and experience in statistics, computer science, logic, and public health.

Crime laboratories—federal, state, and county—employ laboratorians to analyze body fluids, such as blood and semen, as well as other substances from crime-related deaths or injuries. Some laboratorians work directly as FBI investigators or special agents.

State departments of health also employ laboratory scientists to investigate water and air purity, outbreaks of food poisonings, and communicable diseases. A title such as "environment health specialist" may be used for this laboratory professional.

JCAH and CAP are acronyms for the Joint Commission on the Accreditation of Hospitals (now called JCAHO—the Joint Commission on the Accreditation of Healthcare Organizations) and the College of American Pathologists. Both groups inspect laboratories for purposes of accreditation; JCAHO employs laboratorians specifically as laboratory inspectors.

Chapter 5 provides information on career opportunities in the armed services. Altogether, the air force, army, and navy have approximately 450 biomedical laboratory officers and 5000 enlisted laboratory personnel.

Also of interest are opportunities in the U.S. space program. To become a NASA mission specialist astronaut candidate requires a master's degree and two years experience in one's field of interest, such as hematology or immunology, plus other qualifications specified by NASA.

One can also become a patient educator at the local, state, or national level.

In a large hospital or medical center, the opportunities for specialization are great, as demonstrated by 36 entries within this category.

The first category, "andrology," is the study of reproduction, specifically in bringing about the fertilization of ovum and sperm to produce an embryo and then a fetus. Fertility testing and andrology laboratories are most often seen in the reproductive units of medical centers, as laboratorians and scientists attempt to help infertile couples bear children.

The usual laboratory areas of any hospital include blood bank, chemistry, coagulation, hematology, immunology, microbiology, and serology (see appendix A). However, other hospital or medical center laboratory specialty areas include the following:

- **Bone marrow.** Personnel in this area differentiate blood cells formed in the bone marrow, aspirated by bone marrow biopsy, and then stained and examined for normality or malignancy.
- **Cell markers.** Since specific cell proteins on white cells act as antigenic determinants, identification of specific cell types (such as leukemic and lymphoma cells) can be made using monoclonal

antibodies, as well as the markers of heavy and light chains of immunoglobulins.

- **Computer science.** Many laboratories are computerized, using laboratory specialists who write programs, debug packaged programs, and provide the necessary computer interfaces among the laboratory, patient records, and other health professionals.
- **Components/transfusion service.** Since blood can be separated into its components—plasma, red cells, white cells, and platelets—and further fractionated into subcomponents such as factor VIII of plasma, most laboratories offer blood components for transfusion. Experts in component therapy obtain, transport, store, test, and provide blood and its products as needed for surgery, therapy, or prophylactic purposes. Many work not only in hospital laboratories, but also for agencies such as the American Red Cross whose goals include the distribution of safe blood for the community.
- **Cytogenetics.** This is the science of the structure and abnormalities of chromosomes. Laboratory professionals who specialize in cytogenetics usually spend at least six months to one year learning how to grow cells containing chromosomes, separating and grouping chromosomes by position, and locating and identifying abnormalities. The result is a photokaryotype, a picture of the paired chromosomes with specific abnormalities delineated. Cytogenetics is becoming increasingly important in identifying prenatal abnormalities such as Down's syndrome, or disease states such as the leukemias. For example, the "Philadelphia chromosome" is associated with eighty-five percent of patients with chronic myelogenous leukemia.
- **Cytodiagnostic urinalysis** is the subspecialty of urinalysis involving the staining and identification of materials from urinary sediment (the material at the bottom of a centrifuged tube of urine). Special staining helps differentiate urinary crystals, casts, and cells.
- **Cytology and histology** are those areas of anatomic pathology in which body cells and tissues are prepared, stained, and examined for abnormalities. Tissue sections used usually include materials from biopsies, autopsies, and surgeries.

- **Drug analysis,** sometimes called toxicology or drug monitoring, is the chemical science involved in identifying and quantifying drugs in a person's blood, urine, or gastric contents. These drugs may be substances of abuse such as barbiturates, opiates, or amphetamines, or therapeutic drugs such as lithium or digoxin; the latter are measured for a level of therapeutic adequacy, but nontoxicity to the body.
- **Endocrinology.** This chemistry subsection quantitates various hormones, such as insulin, thyroid hormones (T_3, T_4, TSH), cortisol, growth hormone, 17-hydroxyprogesterone, and others.
- **Forensic science.** County, state, and national crime laboratories attempt to determine the cause of death in any case that is not natural. This includes the performance of an autopsy and may also involve blood typing, histocompatibility testing, and other laboratory procedures to help determine not only cause of death but perhaps who might be responsible for one that is criminal in nature.
- **Genetics/genetic counseling.** Specialized genetics laboratories determine not only chromosomal abnormalities but also analyze for errors of inborn metabolism. Thus, specific diseases such as phenylketonuria, tyrosinemia, infant galactosemia, glycogen storage disease, or Tay-Sachs disease may be diagnosed by abnormal levels of various amino acids, organic acids, mono and disaccharides, mucopolysaccharides, and abnormal oligosaccharides. Genetic counseling involves identifying and conferring with persons at high risk for genetic disease in their offspring, so that persons in marriages at high risk may have reproductive options.
- **Immunopathology** involves testing tissue biopsies and blood for pathologic components. Tests include those for DNA, ANA, immune complexes, complement, and components of complement.
- **Infection control** is that area that is concerned with maintaining the institution as free of infectious agents as possible. Investigation is made of nosocomial (hospital-acquired) infections, loss of sterility of usually sterile items or areas, and outbreaks of infections in units such as the nursery. Infection control practitioners usually include laboratorians, nurses, and physicians.

- **Mycology** is a subspecialty of microbiology and involves the identification of fungi that cause cutaneous (skin), subcutaneous (tissue), and systemic diseases. Pathogenic fungi include such examples as *Candida* (a yeast involved in oral thrush); *Hisoplasma,* which causes a lung disease similar to tuberculosis; *Trichophyton,* which causes athlete's foot.
- **Nuclear medicine** has been described in chapter 3. Here, a patient may be given a radioactive substance, such as iodine, and after a short interval, checked for the localization of that radionuclide by way of a scintillation image (an *in vivo* test).
- **Outpatient or clinic laboratories** may be found within a hospital or medical center to provide basic and timely laboratory tests for outpatients.
- **Parasitology** is a subsection of microbiology concerned with the identification of parasites. Examples of parasites include *Plasmodia,* which causes malaria; *Giardia,* which causes diarrhea; *Taenia,* a tapeworm of pork.
- **Pathology** usually includes histology and cytology, jobs which have been described in chapter 3.
- **Phlebotomy/specimen processing.** In many centers, phlebotomists obtain blood samples; these specimens are then processed in a central area. Processing involves separation of serum from red cells; aliquoting serum into smaller samples to be distributed to a number of laboratories; and storing (by refrigeration or freezing) samples that can be batched and tested at specified times.
- **A platelet studies laboratory** is a subspecialty of both coagulation and blood banking and involves testing platelets from patients with drug-induced immune thrombocytopenia (low platelets), posttransfusion purpura (bruising), or autoimmune thrombocytopenia purpura, to determine the reasons for these conditions.
- **Photography/illustration.** Some institutions have their own photographers and illustrators to assist in preparing pictures and illustrations for articles for publication and for education. They also photograph entire specimens and microscopic stained sections of specimens to help diagnose and document abnormalities.

- **Quality assurance (QA).** Certain laboratory personnel may be designated to plan, implement, and oversee quality assurance programs for the laboratory and the institution. To do so, they set standards for the organization, and take corrective action as appropriate. Within a laboratory, QA involves the selection and use of laboratory methods; the performance of tests and reporting of test results; the collection and handling of specimens; the selection, calibration, and maintenance of equipment; the selection and use of reagents, controls, standards, and supplies; the selection, monitoring, and education of personnel; and the development, documentation, use, and review of all testing processes.
- **Skin or bone bank.** Most hospitals have blood banks; a few also have skin banks and bone banks whose products are used in skin grafts (such as for those severely burned) or bone grafts (for those with serious fractures or bone degeneration). The sources of skin and bone are usually cadavers.
- **Special stains.** Personnel in this area perform special stains— cytochemical, fluorescent, and others in order to identify, localize, and study cells and tissues. These stains are used particularly to mark a biochemical process in a particular cell structure.
- **STAT laboratory.** The word STAT means immediately; it is frequently used to identify an emergency laboratory request. Thus, STAT laboratories may be established near areas where emergency situations are frequently encountered: the emergency room, operating room, or neonatal nursery.
- **Tissue typing.** When an organ such as kidney, heart, or pancreas, is transplanted, testing (sometimes called histocompatibility testing) must be performed to determine compatibility between recipient and organ. Most tissue typing involves three kinds of testing: serologic, mixed lymphocyte reactions, and cytotoxic T-cell typing. The intent is the same as for blood transfusions: to minimize rejection of the transplanted organ by matching organ tissue and recipient blood. Tissue typing may also involve HLA (human leukocyte antigen) testing to determine the association between certain white cell antigens and disease.

- **Transplant services.** In association with the blood bank and tissue typing, an institution may also have designated personnel who assist in transplantation procedures. "Perfusionists" (sometimes called extra-corporeal technologists) are skilled persons who maintain a patient's circulatory or respiratory function, usually during surgery. They may also maintain the viability of an organ between the time of removal from the donor to transplantation within the recipient.
- **Virology.** Virology laboratories are found in about ten percent of all hospitals. Personnel there are responsible for identifying the viruses causing acute viral infections as well as determining a patient's immune status to a particular virus (such as polio, measles, mumps). Since viruses will not grow on ordinary laboratory media, they must be grown in tissue culture. Other techniques used in virology vary from tissue culture neutralization to counterimmunoelectrophoresis to hemagglutination inhibition to immunofluorescence and others.

ADMINISTRATIVE POSITIONS

Health care administration includes twenty titles for which laboratory personnel are qualified. To become a laboratory supervisor usually requires experience; to become a director may require an advanced degree, such as a master's, M.B.A., or Ph.D. Other positions are seen on the extended career paths chart, including manager of a clinic or a coder in the business office. Here, one "codes" tests for billing, knowing the nature of the test and the patient's condition. One may also serve as a service specialist, personnel director, coordinator of emergency services (such as a triage coordinator in the emergency room), or financial manager. When doctors get together in a group practice (usually including five or more physicians), one may serve as the overall administrator of that practice.

Since hospitals and all industries are under increasing surveillance for the ways they dispose of waste, some laboratorians are taking positions as coordinators of waste removal, especially hazardous wastes such as needles, syringes, media, specimens, plasticware, and reagents. These hazardous substances are usually first autoclaved (heated to high temperatures with steam under pressure) within the institutions, and then displosed of in appropriate areas. Since laboratory personnel are familiar with potential hazards, they are excellent choices as managers of waste materials disposal units.

With additional training, for example an M.B.A. or Ph.D. degree, one may become an administrator of a hospital, clinic, HMO, as well as an administrator in companies dealing with health insurance or health policy decisions.

Traditionally, coordinators of health promotion programs have come from the profession of nursing or public health. Nevertheless, opportunities are available for laboratorians in health promotion. Laboratory personnel understand what cholesterol is and its derivation, what carbon monoxide (from smoking) does to hemoglobin, as well as the effects of exercise on muscle and its enzymes. Therefore they are excellent resource persons for health promotion programs.

Laboratory quality assurance officers can also go on to become hospital quality assurance coordinators. Likewise, many microbiologists go on to become infection control officers, and with additional course work, epidemiologists (one who is trained to determine the specific cause(s) of an outbreak of infection, or of toxic poisoning, or of any disease of recognized origin). An epidemiologist is also involved in studying the factors determining the frequency and distribution of disease in a population, such as the association of cancer with environmental or industrial carcinogens (agents that cause cancer).

Utilization review (UR) is a form of health care review first carried out in 1965 under the Social Security Act. The intent of utilization review is to ensure the medical necessity and appropriateness of care, and involves the establishment of UR committees to examine inappropriate care. Laboratorians are especially effective in utilization review when they observe misuse of testing (such as ordering too many tests) or inappropriate patterns of testing (such as certain physicians wanting profiles or batteries of tests that are unnecessary).

Finally, within the category of health care administration, a laboratory professional may assume the position of staffing coordinator.

Laboratory practitioners are well known for their organizational abilities; therefore determining staffing patterns (including scheduling and establishing the proper mix of employees) for a unit or institution, is one positive outgrowth.

OTHER OPPORTUNITIES

Management information systems (the management of data through the use of computers and including laboratory information) encompasses five listings ranging from someone who is a computer programmer to one who directs a biometry laboratory.

Health maintenance organizations (HMOs) employ laboratory personnel not only as staff members, supervisors, or directors, but also as administrators.

Laboratorians may also choose to work as consultants, for example in assisting personnel in physician office laboratories in establishing and monitoring quality control, in instrument maintenance, in implementing procedures for safety, and other matters. Other consultantships include those in public health laboratories, clinics, and HMOs.

Other laboratory scientists work in reference or commercial laboratories, where samples are brought for analysis (see chapter 2). These laboratories may specialize in such areas as drug analysis or cytology; representatives may also serve as consultants to assist small laboratories in establishing new procedures, quality assurance, and the like.

Veterinary medicine clinics and zoos employ laboratory scientists to perform hematologic, chemical, microbiologic, and immunologic analyses very similar to those that are available to humans. Sometimes, additional training is needed (for example birds have red cells that are nucleated, humans do not), but most often the equipment, supplies, and reagents seen in veterinary medicine clinics are very similar to those seen in human clinic laboratories. Zoos also employ laboratory personnel whose work is very diverse and challenging, such as in obtaining blood from a lion.

Some laboratorians choose to work abroad, especially in research laboratories, pharmaceutical and product development companies, International Red Cross blood banks, and the like. Some serve as educators, and if involved in humanitarian endeavors (as a missionary or working with the Peace Corps) they may set up laboratories and teach, as well as perform analyses. Project HOPE is devoted to international educational endeavors and uses laboratory professionals as short-term and long-term consultants.

Education is a popular route for laboratorians to take. All 450 NAACLS/CAHEA accredited medical technology programs have a program director or education coordinator in charge. Many universities and health science centers have complete faculties to teach laboratory science. Most of this group have advanced degrees, and they are responsible for teaching, research, and service within their academic units. All other programs, MLT, cytotechnology, nuclear medicine, or specialist in blood bank also require program coordinators who are administrators along with faculty devoted to teaching.

Some laboratory science faculty members go on to become administrators, for example as deans of allied health programs, or as provosts and presidents of colleges and universities.

Other professional routes are attractive as well. Since the laboratory science curriculum is so similar to that completed by premedicine, predentistry, or preveterinary medicine students, lab science graduates often go on to complete these programs as well. Moreover, while in school, these individuals often work part-time in various laboratories, ensuring a good income. Once graduated, baccalaureate-level laboratorians may also choose law, engineering, medical physics or radiation science, optometry (concerning eye examinations and prescriptions), or public health.

In industry, energetic and entrepreneurial laboratory professionals have assisted in developing new tests and equipment, in marketing and selling products, in serving as technical resource persons (troubleshooting problem tests or instruments), and in researching new methodologies. They have also worked for insurance companies, as certified public accountants, as editors or managers of medical publications, in food technology, and in installing equipment. Others work as consultants for the movies or television (one may remember "Quincy").

Finally, research—both basic and applied—attracts some laboratorians (see chapter 2). Researchers may work as technologists, scientists, or as directors of programs.

Not listed on the extended career paths chart, but anticipated in the future, are clinical laboratory professionals serving as independent practitioners. Presently, most laboratory tests are requested by a physician and performed in a physician-directed laboratory. However, with the advent of home testing (pregnancy tests or hand-held glucose analyzers), the locations of laboratory testing are being extended. Moreover, regulations are anticipated which will open the market for testing.

Thus, it can be seen that many and varied job opportunities exist for laboratory professionals. They can choose to study within health care, or move to other endeavors. Nonetheless, their laboratory background suits them well for new opportunities. Clinical laboratory professionals possess concrete scientific and technical skills, organizational abilities, and the follow-through necessary to be successful in any new adventure.

CHAPTER 5

OPPORTUNITIES IN THE ARMED SERVICES

There are three branches of the armed forces that include laboratory personnel: the air force, army, and navy. The following includes some opportunities in each of these service branches.

OPPORTUNITIES FOR UNITED STATES AIR FORCE BIOMEDICAL LABORATORY OFFICERS

Overview

Biomedical laboratory officers in the air force manage, supervise, and perform analyses of biologic and related materials in hospital, environmental/occupational, epidemiological, toxicology, or research and development laboratories. They also teach in medical/clinical laboratory sciences.

Generally, a biomedical laboratory officer manages a medical laboratory or one or more areas of a laboratory located in an air force clinic, small hospital, regional hospital, or medical center. Some officers are assigned to reference laboratories that specialize in performing environmental/occupational, epidemiological, and toxicological analyses. Others are assigned to organizations that are involved in medical research and development. In each instance, they are responsible for the accuracy, precision, and validity of all procedures. Responsibilities include the development of new procedures, staying current in regulatory requirements and scientific developments, and updating of the laboratory with state-of-the-art equipment. Laboratory officers maintain active communications among physicians, nurses, administrators, and other officers to provide effective patient care, and to enhance the capability of the medical service to support its various missions. Formal and informal continued training of medical laboratory specialists (enlisted personnel), is also expected of laboratory officers.

There are currently (1989) 215 biomedical laboratory officers in the United States Air Force.

Wartime Role

Officers will have increased responsibilities in procuring, collecting, storing, and transporting blood and blood products at the Armed Services Whole Blood Processing Laboratory and contingency blood donor centers, as well as each medical treatment facility. The majority of the laboratory officers will be mobilized and assigned to manage laboratories in the prepositioned 500-bed third and fourth echelon combat hospitals. Other laboratory officers will be assigned to each of the hospitals projected as combat casualty treatment centers.

Selection and Specialty Qualifications

CERTIFICATION/REGISTRATION

Those officers working as general laboratory officers are expected to be registered medical technologists with the Board of Registry of the American Society of Clinical Pathologists (ASCP), the National Certifying Agency for Medical Laboratory Personnel (NCA), or an equivalent certifying agency.

ADVANCED DEGREES

A master's/doctoral degree, including the minimum courses required for admission to accredited educational programs for medical technologists, or by the Committee on Allied Health Education and Accreditation (CAHEA), is mandatory for assignment into a specialty or research position. Examples include blood bank, chemistry, toxicology, and microbiology. Officers with subspecialties are expected to seek professional recognition from civilian national certifying boards or agencies such as the American Society for Microbiology, and the American Association for Clinical Chemistry.

EXPERIENCE

A minimum of twenty-four months of experience is mandatory in biomedical laboratory assignments as required for designation as a fully qualified biomedical laboratory officer.

PAY/RANK

Entry-level pay grade is based on a formula offering credit for advanced degrees, certification, and work experience. For example, a new officer who possesses a baccalaureate degree and certification but without work experience, would enter the service as a second lieutenant. A new officer with a doctoral degree, with no certification or work experience, would enter the service as a captain.

Potential Career Paths

Several career paths are available to the biomedical laboratory officer. The most common path for a registered medical technologist laboratory officer is: initial assignment as the clinical laboratory officer of a clinic or small hospital, or section chief or assistant to the department chief within a laboratory at a regional hospital or medical center. Indefinite reserve status (IRS) must be applied for and attained before the second assignment. Successive assignments would include duty as the chief, laboratory services, at larger medical treatment facilities. The second or third assignment could also be an air force-sponsored degree program. Field grade officers receive progressively increasing responsibility in larger facilities, as well as consultant responsibilities.

Specialty trained officers with advanced degrees may also be assigned to research facilities such as the Armed Forces Institute of Pathology, the Armed Forces Radiobiology Research Institute, Clinical Investigation Facilities, or to a specialized laboratory such as the USAF Occupational and Environmental Health Laboratory. Their second or third assignment may be to the Air Force Medical Technology Program (described below) followed by an assignment as a chief, laboratory services. They may also return to a research position.

Some senior officers are assigned to staff positions with the Air Force Surgeon General's office, the Armed Forces Institute of Pathology, the Armed Services Whole Blood Processing Laboratory, the Air Force and Department of Defense Blood Programs, and the Air Force Inspection and Safety Center (Inspector General Team). Officers can also be assigned to Air Force and Tri-Service positions that are responsible for developing and implementing automated systems for the medical service.

All officers have the opportunity to apply for a career-broadening assignment during their careers. The positions that laboratory officers have often occupied are in systems, medical intelligence, recruiting, and as directors of ambulatory services.

The USAF Medical Technology Program

The Air Force Medical Technology Program is a graduate level medical laboratory studies program whose primary purpose is to prepare air force officers to supervise USAF clinical laboratories. Areas of study include medical microbiology, serology, clinical chemistry, hematology, urinalysis, immunohematology, and laboratory management. Course completion qualifies the officer to take the medical technologist certifying examination of the Board of Registry of ASCP, the NCA, or equivalent agencies.

The one-year course is accredited by the Committee on Allied Health Education and Accreditation (CAHEA) in cooperation with the National Accrediting Agency for Clinical Laboratory Sciences (NAACLS). Prerequisites for selection into this graduate level program are:

- Completion of, or in final year of master of science degree from an accredited institution in one of the biological/chemical sciences (chemistry, hematology, virology, toxicology, microbiology) that are acceptable to the Surgeon General, USAF. Active duty personnel or AFROTC cadets may apply with a bachelor of science degree. All other prerequisites must be met.

- Course work must encompass sixteen semester hours (twenty-four quarter hours) of biology to include one semester in microbiology; sixteen semester hours (twenty-four quarter hours) of chemistry to include one semester of organic or biochemistry; and four semester hours in mathematics. Courses in anatomy, genetics, physiology, quantitative analysis, physical chemistry, physics, instrumentation, management, and statistics are recommended.
- Applicants must be physically qualified and eligible for air force commission.
- Civilian applicants apply through the Air Force Recruiting Service.

This graduate level program is located at Malcolm Grow USAF Medical Center, Andrews Air Force Base, Maryland. A maximum of ten interns are enrolled annually.

Career Advancement and Enhancement

Several avenues for career advancement and enhancement are available to the biomedical laboratory officer.

1. Continuing medical education (CME). Officers are expected to have thirty-five hours of CME each year. Fifteen of those hours must be category I or its equivalent. Some CME is available to laboratory officers at their assigned medical treatment facility. Professional laboratory societies on the local, state, and national levels provide meetings periodically for continuing medical education. Usually the laboratory officer is funded by the hospital once per year for national society meetings. Laboratory officers who present scientific papers or posters are usually funded each year to attend the annual meeting of the Society of Armed Forces Medical Laboratory Scientists, at which the opportunity exists to obtain additional continuing education.
2. Tuition assistance for attendance to off-duty education courses (attendance at night classes in pursuit of a Master of Business Administration). These courses are often provided on-base as extension courses through local universities.

3. Air Force Institute of Technology Graduate Education Programs. Based on air force requirements, laboratory officers are selected to attend various civilian institutions for graduate education.
4. Officers are selected annually for fellowships in blood banking, quality assurance, and systems. (The number selected is based on the requirements of the air force.)
5. Formal professional military education (PME) courses prepare officers for advancement within the laboratory field. In addition, PME prepares officers who desire to branch out of the laboratory to enter positions commonly held by administrative personnel in civilian health care facilities.
6. Opportunities for advancement in laboratory management, laboratory education, and specialties (including research) can all be incorporated into the biomedical laboratory officers' career program.

UNITED STATES AIR FORCE MEDICAL LABORATORY SPECIALISTS (ENLISTED PERSONNEL)

Overview

Air force enlisted laboratory technicians (equivalent to medical laboratory technicians) complete a fifty-three-week course in the laboratory sciences. The title of the course is "Medical Laboratory Specialist." It is divided into two segments referred to as phase I and phase II. Provisions are available for proficiency advancement through these courses.

The medical laboratory specialist (phase I) course is seventeen weeks in length. This course is located at the School of Health Care Sciences, Sheppard AFB, Texas. The course encompasses basic theory and skills, collection, preparation, and analysis of biological fluids and other substances by standard procedures used in medical laboratories to aid in the diagnosis, treatment, and prevention of disease. The emphasis is on routine methodologies employed in the fields of urinalysis, hematology, blood banking, immunology, clinical chemistry, bacteriology, mycology, parasitology, medical laboratory automated data processing, and work load reporting. One week of this course is designated for "basic medical readiness."

The medical laboratory specialist (phase II) course is a thirty-six-week course. This course is laboratory-based at several air force medical facilities. Its emphasis is on the fundamental techniques used in a medical laboratory. Students develop an understanding of routine laboratory procedures, and are trained to perform basic laboratory tests with a minimum of supervision. In addition, they gain a knowledge of medical subjects to the extent necessary for their effective performance of duty as medical laboratory specialists.

The mode of instruction for these courses is formal lectures and laboratory (performance) experience.

Educational opportunities available to enlisted members of the air force include, but are not limited to, the following:

- Community College of the Air Force. This community college offers an associate degree for many of the air force specialties.
- Tuition assistance. Assistance is provided to offset the cost of attending off-duty education courses in pursuit of college-level degrees.
- GI bill. This is provided to offset the cost of college education.
- Professional military education. Provided both to enhance personnel retention and advancement.
- Eligibility to apply for the Air Force Medical Technology Program with a bachelor's degree.

Currently there are approximately 1,700 enlisted laboratory personnel assigned to this career field. The number of enlisted in training status is dependent on the number of projected vacancies. During 1988 there were 325 entries into these training programs, with 273 completing phase II.

OPPORTUNITIES FOR CLINICAL LABORATORY
PERSONNEL IN THE ARMY

Army Clinical Laboratory Officer

A medical technologist with a B.S. degree and certification may enter the army as a commissioned clinical laboratory officer, usually as a second lieutenant. The army clinical laboratory officer does not work as a staff technologist, as may be the case for many civilian technologists. Entry-level duties start at the basic supervisory/manager level. Depending on the size of the laboratory to which one is assigned, the army laboratory officer may function as a section supervisor in a large medical center, or as the laboratory manager in a smaller hospital.

The duties of section supervisors or managers are similar to their civilian counterparts, with the exception that the military officer will have other military-specific duties to perform. Generally, the army laboratory officer will be given higher levels of responsibilities and more freedom to carry them out. In addition to being scientifically and technically proficient, the laboratory officer is required to manage personnel, supplies, monies, time, and equipment. An officer will have an active involvement in the budget process, equipment and reagent selection and procurement, personnel training, interfacing with other hospital departments, as well as other managerial functions. Duty performance is important and will be the major criterion for promotion to the next higher officer grade. Medical technologists may expect to rise to the rank of lieutenant colonel over a twenty-year career. A few are promoted to colonel. The initial obligation is three years.

The starting pay ranges from approximately $22,000 to $24,000. Currently, it takes twenty-four months for promotion to first lieutenant and another twenty-four months to captain. Pay exceeds civilian levels quickly, with a captain making $35,000 per year after five years of service. The higher compensation reflects the increased levels of responsibilities and the stresses of military life.

Opportunities exist for advancement and promotion in the Army Medical Service Corps. Advancement is steady and is not dependent upon someone leaving, as may be the case in civilian laboratories. An army officer will change jobs and locations every four to five years, usually moving on to a job of increased responsibility and diversity.

Basic officer courses upon entry, and a twenty-week advanced course after an initial assignment, are required military level courses for army clinical laboratory officers.

To prepare the officer for higher levels of responsibility, both military and civilian training programs leading to a master's degree and/or doctorate are available. Advanced degrees open a wide variety of job opportunities in large medical centers as well as in research and development. The army pays for all educational costs as well as giving the officer his/her regular pay during the training. In addition to basic and advanced officer training courses, a staff and command course is required in military training. A blend of both military and civilian education helps develop the officer into a competent and professional soldier/scientist.

Officers compete with their peers for promotion and education opportunities. Only those having excellent records are chosen. Selection is based on duty performance as well as the needs of the army.

Advantages of the military are job satisfaction, an esprit de corps, a chance to assume increased responsibilities, a wide variety of job and education opportunities, good pay and benefits, and a chance to see different parts of this country and the world.

The Army Medical Department has a full-time active duty force of 115 medical technologists working as clinical laboratory officers around the world.

Army Enlisted Laboratory Specialists

The army trains all of its enlisted medical laboratory specialists (92B) at Fort Sam Houston, San Antonio, Texas. The Laboratory Science Division, Academy of Health Sciences, Fort Sam Houston, has two resident laboratory courses: an entry-level basic course of fifteen weeks duration, and a one-year advanced course. High school graduates with specific academic backgrounds entering the army will attend the initial laboratory course following basic training. This course provides training in entry-level laboratory procedures in chemistry, microbiology, hematology, and blood banking.

Following the basic procedures course, graduates are assigned to a variety of units such as army hospital laboratories, field medical units, or research laboratories. These laboratory specialists are minimally trained and require close supervision, as well as four to six months of on-the-job training (OJT) in order for them to be productive.

After two to three years, medical laboratory specialists return to the Academy of Health Sciences for an advanced laboratory course. Training is provided at a high level. Most who complete the one-year course will work as staff technologists until they become senior enough to assume supervisory responsibilities. The advanced course graduates are well trained and with additional experience make excellent section supervisors.

As enlisted laboratory specialists increase in experience and rank, they may be assigned as laboratory supervisors working directly for the commissioned officer laboratory manager and the chief of the department of pathology. They provide valuable support in such areas as personnel management, supply procurement, budgeting, and other daily laboratory operations. In many areas, the senior enlisted laboratory specialist works under the direct supervision of the chief of the department of pathology.

Enlisted laboratory specialists sometimes acquire college degrees in basic biological and chemical sciences. The scope of practice for the advanced course graduate is comparable to that of the medical technologist. Job opportunities include hospital laboratories, reference laboratories, research laboratories, field hospital laboratories, various administrative staff positions, or academy instructorships.

Currently, there are approximately 1,800 army laboratory specialists assigned to the enlisted laboratory career field. Approximately twenty percent of this force turns over annually, thus requiring an annual training requirement of about 400 basic laboratory students and 120 advanced laboratory students. Enlisted specialists may advance in rank from private (E-1) to sergeant (E-9).

College graduates who are certified medical technologists may also enter the enlisted laboratory field in the grade of E-4 following basic military training, and proceed directly to duty assignment as a medical laboratory specialist. College graduates in biology or chemistry may also enter at the higher grade and work as research assistants in army medical research and development laboratories.

UNITED STATES NAVY OFFICER PROGRAM FOR MEDICAL TECHNOLOGISTS

Description of the Navy Officer Program

Medical technologists commissioned as officers in the United States Navy serve as managers and supervisors of state-of-the-art clinical laboratories in navy hospitals in the United States and many foreign countries. They are integral members of the navy health care team. Additional assignments as educators in navy laboratory schools and investigators in medical research facilities are also available.

Qualified candidates are commissioned to the rank of ensign in the Medical Service Corps. Selection for commissioning is highly competitive. To be competitive for selection, a medical technologist applying for a naval commission must meet the following criteria:

- A Bachelor of Science degree with an overall grade point average (GPA) of at least 3.0.
- Completion of a one year, accredited medical technology training program culminating in a baccalaureate degree, if a degree has not been previously earned.
- Certification as a medical technologist by a national certifying agency upon successful passing of a comprehensive examination.
- A minimum of two years of clinical laboratory experience as a medical technologist.
- Demonstrated leadership and management expertise.
- Evidence of continuing professional education through course work, seminars, workshops, and attendance at professional meetings.

The navy is looking for medical technologists who are leaders and managers, individuals with the background and potential to become strong naval officers. Successful officers are those who can meet the dual responsibility of naval officer and clinical specialist. Navy medical technologists are not bench technologists. They are responsible for directing work of navy enlisted medical laboratory personnel, civilian medical technologists and technicians, and providing professional consultation to the medical staff.

Benefits of the Navy Officer Program

In 1989, the newly commissioned medical technologist earned a minimum starting salary of $21,000. Married officers and those assigned to high cost areas earn more. Pay raises can be expected annually and upon promotion. In 1989 a medical technologist having served ten years on active duty earned a minimum of $41,000 per year. A successful navy medical technologist who is promoted to the rank of captain after twenty years of active duty earned $60,600 in 1989. A medical technologist can retire from the navy after twenty years active service at fifty percent base pay. Retired pay increases 2.5 percent for every additional year of active duty up to 75 percent after thirty years. Therefore, a navy captain retiring after twenty-four years of active duty in 1988 would earn $31,000 a year, with cost of living increases anticipated each year.

In the navy a medical technologist officer joins a very select group of one hundred other medical technologists. They are continually challenged by responsibility and have the opportunity to work in hospitals across the United States and on many foreign shores. These officers look forward to new duty assignments every three to five years, and receive financial rewards greater than those available in the civilian community. Promotion opportunities for navy medical technologists have historically been outstanding and a meaningful navy career and full retirement may be anticipated.

Further information on a career as a navy medical technologist can be obtained from a local navy recruiter or the Navy Specialty Advisor for Medical Technology by calling (202) 295-1562.

NAVY ENLISTED PROGRAM IN LABORATORY MEDICINE

Enlisted personnel play a pivotal role in U.S. Navy medicine as medical laboratory technicians, serving in hospitals and clinics, on board ships, and ashore with the marines.

Navy hospital corpsmen selected to be medical laboratory technicians are provided instruction in the knowledge and skills required to perform and supervise basic and advanced laboratory procedures. Formal training is provided at navy training facilities in Bethesda, Maryland, and San Diego, California.

The one-year course for enlisted personnel includes instruction in clinical bacteriology, mycology, serology, parasitology, hematology, immunohematology, clinical chemistry, toxicology, urinalysis, blood donor processing, and blood banking. Strong emphasis is placed on quality control, record keeping, equipment maintenance, computerization in the clinical laboratory. The course is fully accredited and credits earned are accepted by many colleges and universities.

Prerequisites include enlistment in the U.S. Navy and high school or college courses in algebra and chemistry with grades of "C" or better.

CHAPTER 6

BECOMING A LABORATORY PROFESSIONAL

To become a laboratory professional requires intelligence, a commitment to working hard in school, a desire to help humankind, and a love of science, especially biology. The following is a checklist used in helping to determine whether one is suited to become a clinical laboratory professional.

CHECKLIST

<u>YES</u>   <u>NO</u>

____ ____ 1. It is important to me to have a career that involves helping others.

____ ____ 2. To my friends, family, and teachers, I am known to be a person of honesty and integrity.

____ ____ 3. I have good manual dexterity and can translate thinking skills into doing skills.

____ ____ 4. I like a certain amount of order or structure in the things that I do.

____ ____ 5. I am able to plan and carry out work with little supervision.

<u>YES</u>   <u>NO</u>

____ ____   6. It is important to me to have a sense of accomplishment (achievement) for the work I do.

____ ____   7. In a work situation, I prefer to be busy and use my time well.

____ ____   8. I enjoy problem solving.

____ ____   9. I am capable of working effectively in stressful situations.

____ ____   10. I am able to prioritize and carry out tasks when given several of them to do at the same time.

____ ____   11. I have good communication skills.

____ ____   12. I enjoy using various instruments (such as microscopes) as well as computers.

____ ____   13. I like to know why things happen and what causes certain biologic conditions to occur.

____ ____   14. I enjoy learning new ways of doing things.

____ ____   15. I wish to play a significant role in finding the causes of disease and in helping people to improve their lives.

____ ____   16. I like and do well in science courses, especially biology.

____ ____   17. I know the work in clinical laboratory science involves testing blood and other biological substances for their cellular, chemical, or biological components.

____ ____   18. I understand that with a degree in laboratory science, I can work in laboratories in hospitals, clinics, research, veterinary medicine, industry, and a number of other areas.

____ ____   19. I know that in laboratory science I will use the latest scientific discoveries in my work.

YES   NO

____   ____   20. Following high school, I am willing to spend four to five years (depending on the program chosen) to prepare for a profession in laboratory science.

____   ____   21. Following high school, I would enjoy studying science and other courses needed to prepare for a profession in laboratory science.

____   ____   22. In college, I understand that in order to enter a professional program in clinical laboratory science (medical technology), I will need to demonstrate my academic abilities by earning good grades.

____   ____   23. I understand that a degree in laboratory science/medical technology can be the basis for graduate work in laboratory science as well as in the biological and physical sciences, medicine, dentistry, law, education, and administration, if an advanced degree is desired.

____   ____   24. I know that in some settings, laboratory personnel work with patients with infectious diseases, but that precautions for safety are well established.

____   ____   25. I like medically related activities, but not one hundred percent direct patient contact.

____   ____   26. I understand that laboratory science is a profession based on the team concept in which health care providers work together to achieve positive outcomes.

____   ____   27. I understand that the starting salaries for clinical laboratory personnel are usually comparable to those of other allied health professionals and nurses.

____   ____   28. I recognize that in this profession, I may have to work evening, night, or weekend shifts, depending on the work setting I choose.

____   ____   29. I am willing to treat all patients and their families equally and humanely—with respect and caring.

YES   NO

——   ——   30. As a health care professional, I will be able to keep all patient or client information in the strictest confidence.

(YES)   (NO)   **Total**

To score this assessment instrument, give two points for a yes response to items 2, 3, 5, 8, 9, 10, 12, 16, 17, and 22. These items have been chosen by forty laboratory educators as the ten key statements for a potential student to become a successful laboratory scientist. Give one point to a yes response for each of the other twenty items. If your total score is thirty or more, you are an excellent candidate for becoming a successful clinical laboratory scientist. If you score from twenty to twenty-nine, you are a good candidate. If you score nineteen or less, you should probably investigate other career options.

The checklist can also be grouped in two ways: knowledge of self (items 1–16), and knowledge of the field (items 17–30). Both are important in choosing a career, especially one in laboratory science.

HIGH SCHOOL HIGHLIGHTS

Courses of instruction in a secondary school curriculum are usually measured in terms of *units*. A unit is defined as one year's work on a single subject. Most high school students will study the course of English during each of the four years in attendance thereby accumulating four units in that subject.

For admission eligibility, community and junior colleges, four-year colleges, and universities often require applicants to complete sixteen to twenty units of acceptable high school work. Students considering laboratory science as a career should *not* be enrolled in commercial, vocational, or nonacademic programs of high schools. Enrollment in college preparatory high school curriculums will enhance admission requirements to institutions of higher education.

It is essential that the subject of English be included during each of the four years spent in high school. The ability to read, write, and speak intelligently is increasingly vital to the practice of laboratory science. Future laboratory science students must have a strong foundation in science; they are urged to include the three basic sciences of chemistry, biology, and physics in a high school program. At least two courses in mathematics should be completed, and a student would do well to study the highest level math course consistent with individual ability. As the world grows smaller, knowledge of a foreign language is becoming increasingly important, and three to four units of a language would be helpful.

Completion of English, the sciences, and mathematics as described will yield a minimum of nine of the units needed for collegiate admission. Remaining units may be drawn from courses in social studies, history, and electives. A course in computer science should be considered as one of the elective courses.

What other elective subjects might a high school student select during the secondary school years? Programs in art and music will stimulate an interest in the beauty of sight and sound. Diverse courses are enriching, and the better informed one becomes, the better will be future personal decisions. Subjects such as social sciences, history, and philosophy, provide some investigation of human conduct and principles of being.

A typical high school curriculum that will enhance the chances of one completing a baccalaureate program in laboratory science, includes the following courses:

Courses	Units
English	4
Mathematics	2–3
Biology	1
Chemistry	1
Physics	1
Foreign Language	3–4
Social Studies	2
Electives	4–8
TOTAL	18–24

CURRICULUM A

INTEGRATED PROGRAM. SUGGESTED CURRICULUM SEQUENCE:
QUARTER SYSTEM. NUMBER OF CREDITS ARE IN PARENTHESES.

Fall	*Winter*	*Spring*	*Summer School*
YEAR ONE			
Gen. Chem. (5)	Gen. Chem. (5)	Gen. Biology (5)	
Eng. Comp. (5)	Elective (4-5)	Elective (4-5)	
Math (5)	Elective (4-5)	Elective (4-5)	
MedT Orientation (1)			
YEAR TWO			
Quantitative Analysis (5)	Organic Chem. (5-6)	Organic Chem. (5-6)	
Physics (5)	Physics (5)	Anatomy (5)	
Elective (4-5)	Elective (4-5)	Elective (4-5)	
YEAR THREE			
Biochem. (4)	Biochem. (4)	Math (5) or Statistics (4-5)	
Microbiology (4)	Physiology (5)	Pathology (5)	
Elective (4)	Writing in Science (5)	Elective (4)	
YEAR FOUR/FIVE			
Intro. to Lab Science (2)	Intro to Chem. (5)	Clin. Chem. 2 (6)	Clinical Rotations 20-24 weeks (16-17)
Heme. I (3)	Intro to Clin. Micro. (5)	Immunohematology, Immunology (5)	
Virology, Mycology, Parasitology (3)	Hemostasis/ Instrumentation (3)	Hematology Morphology (4)	
Urinalysis (1)	Management/ Education (1)		
Elective (4-5)			

Total credits needed to graduate: 180

B.S. PROGRAM IN CLINICAL LABORATORY SCIENCE/MEDICAL TECHNOLOGY

The curriculum for becoming a laboratory scientist will vary from institution to institution. However, key courses that usually do not change include those in inorganic and organic chemistry and biology.

CURRICULUM B

3 + 1 PROGRAM. SUGGESTED CURRICULUM SEQUENCE:
SEMESTER SYSTEM. NUMBERS OF CREDITS ARE IN PARENTHESES.

Fall Semester   *Spring Semester*

YEAR ONE

General Chemistry (4)   General Chemistry (4)
English Composition (4)   Anatomy (4)
General Biology (4)   Electives (7-8)
Mathematics (4)

YEAR TWO

Organic Chemistry (5)   Organic Chemistry (5)
Physics (5)   Physics/Instrumentation (5)
Physiology (4)   Elective (4-5)

YEAR THREE

Biochemistry (5)   Immunology (4)
General Microbiology (5)   Computer Science (4)
Histology (5)   Electives (7-8)

YEAR FOUR

Clinical rotations (30 credits) through an accredited hospital program, 50-52 weeks in length. Includes hematology, coagulation, microbiology, chemistry, urinalysis, immunohematology, serology, management, education; some electives such as virology cytogenetics, research.

Total credits needed to graduate: 120

Usual high school prerequisites include biology, chemistry, physics, mathematics, and English. A minimum grade point average of 3.0 (B) should be maintained in high school in order to be successful in a college or university laboratory science program.

It is highly recommended that any prospective student tour a clinical laboratory and interview two to three professionals to obtain information and insights about the field.

For the B.S. degree, two sample laboratory science curricula are shown here; one from the University of Minnesota (A), which is an integrated program and uses the quarter system (eleven weeks = one quarter); the other (B) is from a 3 + 1 program, using the semester system (sixteen weeks = one semester).

One may switch from a quarter to semester system or vice versa easily. To switch credits from the quarter to semester system, divide the number of quarter credits by two-thirds. Therefore, a quarter course of six credits is equivalent to a semester course of four credits ($6 \div 2/3 = 4$). To convert semester credits to quarter credits, one multiplies number of semester credits by one and one-half. Therefore, a two-credit semester course is equivalent to a three-credit quarter course.

It can be seen in curriculum A that students have preclinical courses (year 4, fall, winter, spring quarters) prior to their clinical experience in hospitals. The actual length of time spent in rotations in hospital laboratories is shortened to twenty to twenty-four weeks. In curriculum B, all of the laboratory science professional courses are taught in year 4 in an accredited hospital program. Total length of these rotations is fifty to fifty-two weeks. In some programs, especially those in California, one may need to complete a baccalaureate degree prior to entering a one-year (fifty-week) professional program.

Students interested in laboratory science/medical technology are urged to consult with high school and college advisors who are well informed about various health science curricula, especially math and science prerequisites. If one switches majors, completion of required course work can also be accomplished during evening or summer school, so as to finish prerequisite courses. One should also check periodically with the director of the professional program one is interested in attending, to find out whether changes in the curriculum have been made. (Appendix D lists those accredited laboratory science programs at the baccalaureate level. Other kinds of program listings can be obtained by writing to the Committee on Allied Health Education and Accreditation, AMA, 535 North Dearborn Street, Chicago, Illinois 60610).

To gain entrance to the professional program in laboratory science/medical technology (for example, years 3 or 4 of curriculum A or year 4 of curriculum B), one usually needs a grade point average (GPA) of close to 3.0 or better. Some programs accept minimum grade point averages of 2.5. Admission is usually determined by overall GPA and GPA in prerequisite (science and mathematics) courses. Other factors that may be used by an admissions committee include letters of recommendation, an interview, knowledge of the field as evidenced by an essay, or previous laboratory experience. Usually, however, grade point average is considered as the primary determinant for entrance.

THE PROFESSIONAL PROGRAM

Students in clinical laboratory science are expected to become competent professionals. To do so, they are provided instruction in chemistry, urinalysis, microbiology, blood banking (immunohematology), immunology/serology, hematology, and coagulation. Often student laboratories are used to provide introductory exercises. Other instruction makes use of case studies, computer-assisted materials, demonstrations, discussions, and research methodology.

Clinical rotations refer to the training period of practical experience a student undertakes in a productive laboratory usually located in a hospital. The student is under the supervision of practitioners. This experience is exciting, practical, and rewarding as knowledge and skills learned in the classroom and student laboratory are applied in the real world. During clinical rotations, students also interact with patients and other health care providers. Each day of the clinical rotation adds to the students' self-confidence and moves them closer to becoming real professionals.

PERSONAL ATTRIBUTES

The thirty-item checklist found earlier in this chapter includes some of the personal characteristics that will enhance one's chances of becoming a successful practitioner who enjoys his or her work.

Firstly, an interest in science is very important. Of all high school courses completed, biology is probably the most important. In fact, many professionals believe that an interest and success in biology is more important than an interest and success in chemistry, physics, or mathematics. Nevertheless, one who is interested in biologic as well as medical phenomena will be well suited for this profession.

Secondly, one must be of the highest personal integrity. Accurate laboratory information is crucial to the health and well-being of individuals; thus, the mislabeling of tubes or specimens, careless work, or reporting erroneous results cannot be tolerated. Professionals and students must also be able to say, "I made a mistake," and go about correcting it.

Thirdly, one must be a good student—intelligent, hardworking, motivated; one who does not put off studying. As in medicine, we in laboratory science want the brightest and the best; therefore, achieving a good grade point average is important.

Fourthly, one should have good manual dexterity—the ability to manipulate test tubes, reagents, microscopes, and instruments such as computers in a skillful manner. The person who is known as a "klutz" may not be suited for a laboratory career, although one's manual dexterity usually improves with experience and confidence.

Fifthly, one should be able to prioritize—to attend to matters that require immediate action, and to be able to decide upon other concerns that can be carried out later. Patient care is not predictable; often, one can receive three STAT requests simultaneously. Thus the laboratorian who can sort out the importance of each and complete the work well and in a timely fashion is one of the most valued members of the health care team.

Similar to the above attribute, is the ability to work under stress—a person who is "turned on" by the immediacy of a STAT situation, who can remain calm and productive when physicians and nurses are being demanding, and who can communicate with others when they are less than courteous, will find laboratory science exciting and meaningful.

A person who is considering this profession should also be able to plan and carry out tasks with very little supervision. Laboratorians are known for their sense of independence—for being able to analyze a situation and, on their own, go about completing any work that needs to be done. Coupled with many of the previous attributes is an enjoyment of problem solving. If a person gains a sense of satisfaction in fixing things, he or she will be much sought after in the laboratory; if able to troubleshoot instruments, this person will be extremely valued.

Finally, when one considers that, for example, a ten-year career involves 20,800 hours of employment, it is essential that the person interested in laboratory science understand the field, the course work and grades required to complete the program, as well as the opportunities available upon graduation. Thus, the inquisitive student who visits two or three laboratories, talks to a number of professionals, and visits several accredited educational programs will have an advantage over those who are somewhat interested, but not as aggressive. Note, however, that many laboratory scientists have started in school in other majors; once they have become familiar with the field, they then switch into it. That, too, is acceptable, since many young adults find their niche not in year one of school, but later on.

The checklist provides information on other personal characteristics that are important: a desire to help others, to have a sense of accomplishment for work done well, to have good communication skills, to be curious, to enjoy learning new things, to use cutting-edge technologies, to be motivated, and to have carry through.

A potential laboratory science student should also understand the nature of laboratory work. A student may volunteer to assist in a laboratory; in this way he or she will gain knowledge of the field as well as the atmosphere in which it is practiced. It is also important for a student to understand the many settings (see chapter 2) as well as the positive and negative aspects of working in these settings. Finally, one should obtain figures on salaries and benefits—which do vary by region—so as to understand the financial rewards in becoming a laboratory professional.

From the above, one might conclude that the laboratory science profession demands smart, motivated, and caring individuals. This is true—but as health care providers, laboratory professionals can be nothing less.

Listed next are a recent graduate's ten rules for survival for a student enrolled in a clinical laboratory science program. From a student's perspective, these rules also reinforce the necessity for character traits of honesty, integrity, and fair-mindedness.

TEN RULES FOR SURVIVAL IN
LABORATORY SCIENCE EDUCATION

Written By Janice L. Putnam, B.S. Medical Technologist, recent graduate, University of Minnesota.

1. Be honest with yourself and others.

The career you have chosen is one that requires personal integrity and absolute honesty. As a medical technologist, you will be part of a patient care team. It will be your responsibility to perform accurate laboratory tests and interpret them carefully, so that physicians and other health care workers can determine an appropriate course of patient treatment. If honest work is your policy while in school, it will carry over into your work as a practicing laboratorian. Copying or cheating in school is, of course, dishonest, and may be grounds for dismissal. However, as a medical technologist, cheating is much more serious, because it will be harmful to the well-being of a patient. Always think of your work as providing a service for others. Make a commitment to give the same quality service to patients that you would expect to receive as a patient.

2. Practice respect for your fellow classmates.

You and your classmates are pursuing a mutual goal—graduation in the field of medical technology. Along the way, you will spend numerous hours together in lecture, in laboratories, and between classes. Some of you will become close friends. Others will not share the same closeness. Each student, however, is unique and any differences among students should be respected. Competition, jealousy, and other personal conflicts benefit no one. As a professional, you will also have contact with people from varied backgrounds and personalities. If you learn to respect the differences among your classmates, you will be more kind, gentle, and caring of both the patients and other health care providers you will work with as a medical technologist.

3. Never hesitate to ask for help from your instructors.

The information presented in lectures and practiced in the laboratory is sometimes intense. It may be difficult to comprehend the details, even when reviewing lecture notes and laboratory experiments after class. The main goal of instructors is to educate qualified medical technologists. If you do not understand the material presented, make an appointment to see the instructor. No question is too trivial, and most instructors will gladly take the time to help you understand.

4. **Budget your time wisely.**
The high cost of a college education leaves most students with no choice but to work, in addition to attending classes and studying. Wise utilization of each day is important for successful completion of a program. If outside work is a financial necessity, try to find a job with some flexibility, so that as class schedules change, you can adjust your work schedule accordingly. Attending classes, finishing assigned homework, and studying should be your primary priority. While it is important to be financially secure, do not allow outside employment to jeopardize your ultimate goal.

5. **Take care of your health.**
The demands of college course work can be exhausting. It is important to take care of your health in order to function at your fullest capacity. A healthy diet, regular exercise, and an adequate amount of sleep will keep you alert and energetic enough to meet the challenges of the medical technology program.

6. **Always view new information with a questioning mind.**
A medical technologist is a scientist. A scientist learning new information should want to know not only what it means, but also how it came about, and how it can be expanded upon. As a medical technology student, you will be presented with new material every day. Rather than just memorizing the "facts" for an exam, question what you have learned. Discuss it with fellow students and with your instructors. Expand upon it. Success and personal satisfaction in your career will come about if you learn to think as a scientist.

7. **Listen to upperclass students, but use your own best judgment.**
Whether or not you choose to accept upperclassmen's words as sacred should be determined by your own experiences. An unpleasant experience or encounter for one student is hardly reason for others to form prejudices. Enter every class and meet every new instructor with an open mind. Then, based on your own experiences, you may agree or disagree with the opinions of upperclass students.

8. Never stop learning.

Medical technology is an ever-changing profession with newer methods, better technology, and increasing responsibilities. It is imperative that as a graduate you continue to learn so that you may progress further in your profession. Continuing education may be the farthest thought from your mind while an undergraduate. However, you must think ahead toward directions that will broaden your future as a professional.

9. Take time for fun.

Extracurricular enjoyment is essential for one's mental and physical health. While it is important to put forth your best effort as a student, it is impossible to learn every detail. Sometimes you need to take a break. Go to a movie, have dinner with a friend, engage in a hobby or sports activity you enjoy, or sit back and watch TV. Relax your mind when the need arises. You will then be better able to enjoy learning.

10. Act as a professional.

The first nine rules are guides toward becoming a professional. Integrate them into your life. Do not ignore laboratory test results that are out of the control range, or do not make sense. Learn how to resolve these and other problems. Treat all patients humanely by putting aside personal matters or prejudices that might otherwise interfere. Keep yourself well-groomed, well-mannered, and able to get along with others. Keep up to date on the latest advances in diagnostic medicine. Practice the knowledge and skills you have acquired in order to assure quality patient care, and always act as a professional medical technologist.

APPLYING TO A LABORATORY SCIENCE PROGRAM

Once a student has decided on a program in laboratory science, he or she should apply to that program and perhaps two or three others as well. In a large college or university the application may mean completing an application form and submitting a transcript. In a hospital-based program, one may need to submit the above, plus letters of recommendation. It is important that the applicant fill in all forms neatly and completely, since these are the first pieces of information about him or her that members of an admissions committee will see.

Most applications require submission of an application fee; be sure to include a check or money order in the right amount, made payable to the institution. Some organizations hold the application and will not act on it until the check is in receipt. It is best to follow these directions: (1) make the check payable to the institution's name (not to the name of the admissions officer); (2) make certain the amount of the check is equal to the application fee; (3) be sure to mail the check together with the application in the same envelope; and (4) make certain your checking account has sufficient funds to cover the check.

Once an admissions committee has received all credentials, the applicant may be invited for an interview. The interview provides the applicant an opportunity to visit the program directly. Even if an interview is not required, the applicant should make it a point to personally visit a program prior to commitment of attendance. The interview, though considered an evaluation tool by some, is really a mutual instrument of communication that serves to permit direct transmission of information helpful to the admission procedure. During the interview, it is important that the applicant be dressed neatly, poised, confident, and sincere.

Evaluation tools available to an admissions committee include transcripts, test scores, letters of recommendation, and interview encounters. Unquestionably the transcript is the most important and reliable tool of all. To an admissions committee, the transcript represents a totality of grades earned by one student over a period of time from many instructors. Thus, it will be used most extensively to evaluate the applicant's potential.

If an applicant is accepted to a program, he or she should write promptly to the institution, informing the program director of his or her intent to attend. Thereafter, the program director will inform the student of starting dates and any other admissions or orientation information.

LICENSURE/CERTIFICATION

Once a health care professional completes a program of study, he or she usually takes a licensure or certification examination. The first is required by law; the second is voluntary but strongly recommended and often is required by employers. The purpose of each kind of credential—License or certificate—is that of a gatekeeper, to prevent incompetent persons from practicing. Licensure and certification are instituted to help protect the public health, safety, and welfare.

Dentists, nurses, pharmacists, and physicians are usually licensed to practice in the state in which they provide their services. Licensure is the process by which a government or agency grants permission to persons meeting predetermined qualifications to engage in a specific occupation. Usually these predetermined qualifications include completion of a professional program and passing of a state licensure examination. If one is not licensed, he or she cannot legally practice in that state.

In laboratory science, licensure is not the primary mode of gatekeeping, except in a few states and New York City. Successful passing of a state licensure examination is required for laboratory professionals to practice in California, Tennessee, and Florida. Personnel licensure also exists in Georgia, Hawaii, Nevada, North Dakota, and West Virginia, but does not require passing of a separate state licensing exam.

In laboratory science, most graduates take certification examinations. Certification is the process by which a nongovernmental agency or association grants recognition to an individual who has met predetermined qualifications—usually passing a certification examination—specified by that agency or association. Certification is voluntary; one does not legally need a certificate to practice. However, most graduates of laboratory science programs take certification examinations, since employers strongly recommend or require that employees hold a certificate.

Certification in laboratory science is complex and confusing, since there have been five agencies involved in providing certification examinations. A brief review of the two major agencies is provided.

Board of Registry of the American Society of Clinical Pathologists (ASCP)

In 1928 the ASCP established the Registry of Technicians to register individuals who met certain requirements in training and education. The first certificates given required graduation from high school or a diploma from a school of nursing and one year of training. In 1933, applicants were required to pass an essay examination and an oral and practical (hands-on) examination before certification was granted. In 1934, educational requirements were increased to two years of college including science courses, and one year of clinical training. This 2 + 1 pattern continued until 1962, when these requirements were replaced by three years of college and one year of clinical experience. The late 1960s and 1970s saw the rise of 2 + 2 baccalaureate programs, primarily in large colleges and universities, in addition to traditional 3 + 1 programs.

In 1963, ASCP began providing certification examinations for laboratory technicians. The Board of Registry of ASCP has also certified individuals other than generalists: cytotechnologists, histotechnologists, histologic technicians, technologists in chemistry, hematology, immunology, microbiology, and nuclear medicine, as well as specialists in blood banking, chemistry, hematology, immunology, and microbiology. By the close of 1988, the Board of Registry had certified 283,277 individuals, including 178,097 medical technologists.

National Certification Agency for
Medical Laboratory Personnel (NCA)

In 1977 the American Society for Medical Technology helped to establish a new certification agency, independent of control by any professional association. Prior to that time, the Board of Registry, under the auspices of ASCP, controlled the certification of the majority of laboratory personnel. Many laboratory professionals chafed under the ASCP arrangement, and through their efforts initiated NCA. In 1978 NCA offered its first examinations for two generalist categories: the category of clinical laboratory scientist (CLS) and that of clinical laboratory technician (CLT). Other examinations are now available, including those in management, in specialty areas such as cytogenetics, and in phlebotomy.

Many laboratory personnel believe that NCA best represents their interests as the preferred certifying body. NCA has gained in reputation, primarily because of the excellence of its examinations, which are based on competence statements of actual practice in the laboratory. Moreover, NCA seeks recertification of its certificants—either through completion of continuing education credits, or through retesting. NCA is thus committed to continuing competence, not just initial certification. Whether NCA will ultimately be the preferred certification agency, will be seen with time. By the close of 1988, less than eleven years after its inception, NCA had certified 60,000 laboratory personnel, either through certification by examination, or through recognition of prior credentials.

Other Agencies

Three other agencies also provide certification examinations:

AMERICAN MEDICAL TECHNOLOGISTS (AMT)

In 1939 a group of laboratory personnel founded AMT, a certification agency used mainly by graduates of proprietary schools. In addition, AMT also approves laboratory education programs through the Accrediting Bureau of Health Education Schools. AMT certification requirements focus on technical training and work experience. Its medical technologist examination can be taken by persons with a baccalaureate degree as well as by AMT technicians with three years of experience. Members of AMT have tended to be graduates of one- or two-year proprietary schools who first qualified for the technician category and then, with work experience and passing of the AMT technologist's examination, gained medical technologist (MT) status. The AMT has an active registrant list of approximately 18,000.

INTERNATIONAL SOCIETY FOR CLINICAL LABORATORY TECHNOLOGY (ISCLT)

Founded as a splinter group of AMT, ISCLT is a professional society of laboratory personnel with a membership composed primarily of persons trained on the job (OJTs). ISCLT also began providing a certification examination in 1962 through its credentialing commission; its present efforts are directed to the medical technologist (RMT) and laboratory technician (RLT) categories. ISCLT examinations are available to persons who have had experience in the laboratory and who are sponsored by a supervisor. By the close of 1988, ISCLT had an active membership list of approximately 10,000.

DEPARTMENT OF HEALTH AND HUMAN SERVICES (HHS)

To further complicate certification efforts, the federal government began proficiency examinations for supportive-level personnel in 1975. The intent of these examinations was to ensure that the independent laboratories that performed testing for Medicare patients had sufficient "properly qualified technical personnel." At that time many independent laboratories employed numerous supportive-level personnel but fewer persons holding degrees. Since Medicare requirements for reimbursement were quite stringent—for example, that a supervisor be in attendance while supportive-level personnel were working—many independent laboratories and hospital laboratories as well, did not meet Medicare standards. The Department of Health, Education and Welfare (HEW), now HHS, tried to upgrade the status of workers employed through examination, rather than downgrade its original standards. Many supportive personnel outside of independent laboratory settings took the HEW examinations in an attempt to gain status, and perhaps to prepare for further governmental regulations. Over fifty thousand supportive-level personnel and cytotechnologists from a variety of laboratory settings have taken the HEW examinations. Approximately one-half have passed and have been certified by HEW as clinical laboratory technologists or cytotechnologists. Contact the Department of Health and Human Services in Washington, D.C., for information on the status of the HHS proficiency test for medical technologists.

GRADUATE PROGRAMS

Clinical laboratory scientists are well prepared to enroll in graduate programs, both at the master's and doctoral levels. Their backgrounds suit them well for advanced degrees. Examples of programs for which they may enroll include but are not limited to the following:

- Anatomy
- Biochemistry
- Biomedical engineering
- Biometry
- Business administration
- Cell biology
- Clinical chemistry
- Clinical laboratory science
- Computer and information systems
- Education
- Environmental health
- Epidemiology
- Genetics
- Health informatics
- Hematology
- Hemostasis
- History of medicine
- Immunohematology
- Immunology
- Laboratory medicine
- Management
- Microbial engineering
- Microbiology
- Molecular biology
- Pathology or pathobiology
- Pharmacology
- Physiology
- Public health
- Virology

Students may also find areas of interest within other graduate programs. Thus, a specialization in hematology may be found within a department such as anatomy. An immunology concentration might be found in pathobiology, or an epidemiology emphasis with a school of public health.

Undergraduate (baccalaureate level) students who wish to obtain an advanced degree should take the Graduate Record Examination (GRE) close to the time of graduation, when course work is still very familiar.

Finally, *Peterson's Guides* (found in every medical library) list the programs and schools which offer advanced degrees.

CHAPTER 7

ISSUES FOR THE PROFESSION
AND THE PRACTITIONER

INTRODUCTION

Every profession changes and evolves, or dies. For example, physician Paul Starr recently published a book about the various changes that the medical profession has experienced in its history. Many of those changes are now being experienced by the allied health professions. These changes include moving from little if any regulation by state or federal goverment, to considerable regulation by both; changes in how the profession certifies its practitioners; and changes that have to do with how one profession comes to compete with another to deliver health care and be reimbursed for it. Competition—who can compete with whom to do what—is often determined by what are known as "scope-of-practice" definitions. These are generally contained in state or federal laws, such as state practice or licensure acts, or the federal laws creating Medicare.

Clinical laboratory science is going through changes like these today in relation to medicine (particularly to pathology), and to a lesser extent, to nursing, and to certain allied health professions. They are taking the form of issues that must be resolved, first within each profession through the process of building consensus, and later, between or among the professions involved.

These issues are just as important for the professional to master as the solid scientific technical principles underlying his or her field. They have an enormous influence on what professionals do every day; whether they will be allowed to expand their roles and duties as new technology and new insights broaden their competence, and how much gratification they will derive from their profession.

This chapter focuses on a few of the main issues with which today's clinical laboratory professionals are grappling. They are professional independence; health care cost containment and laboratory reimbursement; and future changes in practice patterns. You can see that it is quite an exciting time to be a clinical laboratory science professional!

THE STRUGGLE FOR PROFESSIONAL INDEPENDENCE

One of the most interesting aspects about contemporary health care is the inevitable struggle being waged by the so-called allied health professions for independence from medicine. In other words, like nursing, many of the allied health professions began as helping occupations subordinate to medicine. Early practitioners performed routine tasks and errands assigned by doctors.

However, changes in science, technology, and social mores, coupled with new insights into human health care needs and capabilities and, lately, unprecedented pressures on the health care delivery system, have combined to advance these old "helping occupations" to their status today as professions, or near-professions. With that giant step has come allied health professionals' understandable desire to practice to the full extent of their professional competence. As their competence has expanded, however, it has inevitably brought these practitioners from a position as subordinates of doctors to colleague status, creating tensions over professional territory and compensation.

The issues at stake are basically how the two fields, pathology and clinical laboratory science, will interact in the future, and whether clinical laboratory science will gain full autonomy from pathology. The struggle began over fifty years ago; just how far clinical laboratory science has come can be seen in a quick history of the field and in how its statements, or codes, of professional ethics have evolved.

A BRIEF HISTORY OF CLINICAL LABORATORY SCIENCE

M. Ruth Williams, an early historian of the profession, gives several possibilities for how clinical laboratory science began. One possibility, which she attributes to Vivian Herrick, a medical technologist writing in 1937 in the *American Journal of Medical Technology,* is that it can trace its beginnings to 1550 B.C., when certain intestinal parasites were mentioned in writing. Another is that in the 14th century, in Bologna, Italy, a young woman named Alessandra Giliani served as the first medical technologist. She was employed, we're told, with a physician at the university of Bologna "performing certain tasks which would now be considered those of the technologist," and died from a laboratory-acquired infection—most unlikely today!

Others, however, prefer to date the profession much later, in the 1600s. According to Herrick:

Malpighi (1628–1694) is described as the greatest of the early micros-copists and his work in embryology and anatomy definitely marks him as the founder of pathology.

Others date the founding of laboratory science "with Schwammerdam's discovery of red blood corpuscles," or at 1683, with Leeuwenhoeck's refinement of the microscope lens and pioneering description of blood cells, protozoa, and bacteria. And some prefer a later date still, linking the profession's origins to Pasteur and Koch and their advances in bacteriology (1876), or to Virchow (1821–1902) who specialized in cellular physiology and who is credited with having founded the Archives of Pathology in Berlin, in 1847.

Williams believes the first "chemical laboratory" related to medicine in the United States was founded at the University of Michigan at some time close to 1844. A laboratory assistant at that time (later to become a physician and dean of the Michigan College of Medicine) described some of his work:

I remember with what pride I demonstrated leukemic blood and urine to the class; how I exhibited crystals of tyrosin and leucin in the urine in a case of cancer of the liver, a rare opportunity indeed; how I showed the presence of urea in the perspiration of a man dying of kidney disease. (Vaughan)

Though some of the procedures he describes are routine today, Vaughan nevertheless captures an excitement that still is felt when a clinical laboratory professional detects an important diagnostic clue. Before long, the new field was launched:

One of the first official references to laboratory workers is found in the 1900 census which listed 100 technicians, all male, employed in the United States. These were not all medical technicians, but included some dental and industrial workers. The number of technicians had increased to 3,500 by 1920, with 2,000 of these female. . . . [By] 1922, 3,035 hospitals reported they had clinical laboratories. (Williams)

Gradually, Williams tells us, the demand grew for appropriately trained laboratory technicians. Sometime around 1922 or 1923, the first baccalaureate program in medical technology was founded at the University of Minnesota. Shortly thereafter, the American Society of Clinical Pathologists (ASCP), an organization of pathologists who employed technicians, established certain qualifications for technicians, and created a Board of Registry to certify individuals who met them to practice as medical technologists. By 1933, however, some technicians recognized the need for their own professional association. With the founding that year of the forerunner of the American Society for Medical Technology, the long struggle for professional independence had begun.

In the early 1900s, medical technologists and technicians performed routine functions always under the supervision of the pathologist laboratory director, and all laboratories were in hospitals to serve the needs of hospital patients. However, soon after World War I, pathologists recognized that laboratory services were also needed for physician's patients outside the hospital, and they created outpatient laboratories to serve that need. However, things began to change.

Until the 1930s, the ownership and operation of clinical laboratories, whether in or out of the hospital, were exclusively the domain of pathologists, who had long considered that providing clinical laboratory test results was within "the practice of medicine." However, enterprising clinical laboratory scientists, initially based in California, formed competing laboratories. . . .

In 1940, competent persons holding Ph.D.s, such as clinical chemists and bacteriologists, won the right to be licensed in California as laboratory directors. (Karni et al., *Clinical Laboratory Management*, 1982.)

The challenge was issued, and the struggle over whether clinical laboratory science is or is not part of the practice of medicine began in earnest, with obvious stakes. If it were, then competent nonphysicians would be limited forever in the duties and functions they could legally perform. If it were not, they could legally and competently own, direct, and operate laboratories in any setting.

The use of automated test technologies in the 1950s and the creation of the Medicare and Medicaid programs in the 1960s, raised the stakes and intensified struggle between pathology and clinical laboratory science. Automated multichannel test instruments meant that huge volumes of samples could be tested quickly, cheaply, and usually reliably. And Medicare and Medicaid programs created in 1965, transformed the federal government into a major purchaser of laboratory services for the elderly and the needy, stimulating a huge demand for health care services that has still not been fully contained. The question of laboratory ownership, direction, and control became a struggle between elements of organized pathology and nonphysican clinical laboratory practitioners, with the real issues—professional autonomy and access to compensation for services within one's scope of practice—often buried beneath unjustified challenges of the nonphysician's competence and qualifications to serve in directoral roles. (Bailey, White)

The struggle continues today. Significant gains have been made by clinical laboratory scientists, including agreement by certain state attorneys general and the U.S. Department of Health and Human Services (HHS), that clinical laboratory science is *not* part of the practice of medicine, upheld by the U.S. Court of Appeals. But the dispute has not yet been fully resolved, and will certainly continue for the foreseeable future as necessary changes are sought in three realms:

1. *Private sector hospital and laboratory accreditation standards.* In some instances, personnel qualifications embedded in standards for the accreditation of hospitals or laboratories may be used unfairly, to bar clinical laboratory scientists from serving as hospital laboratory directors.
2. *State personnel licensure laws.* At this writing, only eight states license clinical laboratory personnel and, therefore, determine their scope of practice. However, at least fifteen states are seeking licensure.
3. *Medicare and other key federal laboratory-related laws and regulations.* Personnel standards enacted by the federal government to help determine whether a laboratory can be paid for services to Medicare beneficiaries by Medicare and Medicaid are being extensively revised at this writing. Although Medicare and Medicaid have always permitted qualified nonphysicians to direct hospital and independent laboratories and will certainly continue to do so, standards requiring certain education and experience qualifications for supervisory and staff technologists and technicians have been proposed for elimination. If that occurs—over the strongest objections of all clinical laboratory professional associations—new problems affecting the professional status of clinical laboratory science could arise.

PROFESSIONAL ETHICS

A great deal can be learned about the growth of the profession from a comparison of its various codes of ethics. Codes of ethics, after all, address what the members of a profession believe are its defining characteristics, the functions and roles that distinguish them from all others.

In 1961, ASMT adopted this code of ethics for its members:

Being fully cognizant of my responsibilities in the practice of Medical Technology, I affirm my willingness to discharge my duties with accuracy, thoughtfulness, and care.

Realizing that the knowledge obtained concerning patients in the course of my work must be treated as confidential, I hold inviolate the confidence placed in me by patients and physicians.

Recognizing that my integrity must be pledged to the absolute reliability of my work, I will conduct myself at all times in a manner appropriate to the dignity of my profession. (ASMT)

Thirty years or so ago, the practice of medical technology as perceived even by members of the first autonomous professional association, was simply a matter of accuracy, confidentiality, reliability, and dignity—all essential behaviors, but behaviors that should characterize any professional. That early code really pertained to a supporting practitioner; it simply did not address the duties a true profession would impose on its members.

Today, the ASMT Code of Ethics as revised in 1988 describes a much different professional, this one with clear responsibilities in the laboratory, to the patient, to the profession, and in the community at large.

CODE OF ETHICS OF THE ASMT

Preamble

The Code of Ethics of the American Society for Medical Technology (ASMT) sets forth the principles and standards by which clinical laboratory professionals practice their profession.

The professional conduct of clinical laboratory professionals is based on the following Duties and Principles:

I. Duty to the Patient

Clinical laboratory professionals are accountable for the quality and integrity of the laboratory services they provide. This obligation includes continuing competence in both judgment and performance as individual practitioners, as well as in striving to safeguard the patient from incompetent or illegal practice by others.

Clinical laboratory professionals maintain high standards of practice and promote the acceptance of such standards at every opportunity. They exercise sound judgment in establishing, performing, and evaluating laboratory testing.

Clinical laboratory professionals perform their services with regard for the patient as an individual, respecting his or her right to confidentiality, the uniqueness of his or her needs and his or her right to timely access to needed services. Clinical laboratory professionals provide accurate information to others about the services they provide.

II. Duty to Colleagues and the Profession

Clinical laboratory professionals accept responsibility to individually contribute to the advancement of the profession, through a variety of activities. These activities include contributions to the body of knowledge of the profession; establishing and implementing high standards of practice and education; seeking fair socioeconomic working conditions for themselves and other members of the profession; and holding their colleagues and the profession in high regard and esteem.

Clinical laboratory professionals actively strive to establish cooperative and insightful working relationships with other health professionals, keeping in mind their primary objective to ensure a high standard of care for the patients they serve.

III. Duty to Society

Clinical laboratory professionals share with other citizens the duties of responsible citizenship. As practitioners of an autonomous profession, they have the responsibility to contribute from their sphere of professional competence to the general well-being of the community, and specifically to the resolution of social issues affecting their practice and collective good.

Clinical laboratory professionals comply with relevant laws and regulations pertaining to the practice of clinical laboratory science, and actively seek, within the dictates of their consciences, to change those which do not meet the high standards of care and practice to which the profession is committed.

(Reprinted with permission of the American Society for Medical Technology.)

One of the most enlightening phrases in the 1988 ASMT Code of Ethics is this one: "Clinical laboratory professionals actively strive to establish cooperative and insightful working relationships with other health professionals...." It seems to suggest a peer, or collegial, relationship among clinical laboratory professionals and all other health care practitioners, including physicians. That, of course, is the first step along the path of healthy competition.

HOW LAW AND REGULATION AFFECT THE PROFESSION

ASMT's 1988 Code of Ethics explicitly recognizes the duty of the professional to address laws and regulations affecting the practice. That is because, as we've just seen, these documents can have more influence on the life of the profession and its practitioners than any other development except perhaps technological change.

Today, federal, state, and local laws and regulations influence every facet of the profession. Some influence who may perform clinical laboratory services; some determine how a large share of them shall be paid; others mandate safety precautions to protect the practitioner, and others establish quality assurance safeguards to protect the patient, to name just a few of the issues they address.

In fact, a great deal of what takes place every day in the laboratory occurs at least partly because of federal, state, or local governmental requirements. Laboratory practitioners themselves carry out the quality control, record-keeping, hiring, safety, and other requirements of law or regulation both because these functions generally are good practice, and because they are responsible for ensuring compliance with such requirements.

Drug testing gives an example of how the federal government affects daily practice in the laboratory. Who performs drug testing; what drugs are involved; what minute quantities of each (or threshhold concentrations) will be detected; and what technical procedures, quality control, security, and confidentiality safeguards are imposed on the specimen collection, handling, and testing process are among the issues addressed in federal regulations concerning drug testing for military and certain federal civilian personnel.

Taken as a whole, federal, state, and local laws and regulations govern the laboratory facility, its personnel, many of its technical procedures, and its quality assurance practices. Federal law and regulations also provide civil rights protections and antidiscrimination safeguards for employees; set up procedures for labor disputes; regulate new medical devices, blood, and blood products; and influence a great many other aspects of laboratory practice.

More important in some ways, however, federal regulations especially influence the profession, the practitioner, and the public in other ways that are perhaps more profound but not necessarily as evident.

For instance, as we saw in the preceding discussion about the struggle for professional independence, state and federal laws and regulations that establish mandatory educational and experience requirements for laboratory directors, supervisors, and staff may do more than influence the quality of testing the patient receives. Intentionally or inadvertently, fairly or unfairly, wisely or otherwise, personnel standards can encourage or discourage competition between groups of qualified practitioners. By determining who can play what role, they ultimately can affect the cost and even the availability of laboratory services.

Some regulations can manipulate broad economic forces in such a way as to benefit some laboratories and not others. Some can encourage or discourage certain health care practices, types of testing, or testing devices that can affect the kinds of tests available. They can also send "messages" that infuence whether and how the manufacturing industry will develop and design new technologies, and whether and how new professional career paths will evolve. Federal policy on organ transplantation is an example of the way in which a federal initiative helped to promote histocompatibility testing, a laboratory specialty.

And so it is with other types of regulation, for the laboratory and other health care professions. Because federal and state regulations (1) have the force of law and carry penalties for noncompliance; (2) have broad effect; and (3) address sweeping issues such as the quality, cost, and availability of health care services, they are extremely powerful and extremely complex forces in the health care marketplace. This is not to say that there should be none. The intent of most regulations specific to the clinical laboratory performance is to improve the quality of laboratory services in order to protect the public. For the most part, they have accomplished those goals.

Studies have shown that laboratories that comply with sound standards governing the qualifications of personnel and the quality of the data collected, and also that participate in a process known as "proficiency testing" have lower error rates than those that do not.

But even when they lead to good ends, federal and state laws and regulations can have other consequences. Simply put, what the federal government does and does not do to regulate the quality, cost, and availability of health care generally, and clinical laboratory services particularly, will probably have a greater impact on the clinical laboratory professional than any other force except science and technology.

For these reasons, practicing professionals must have a thorough understanding of government's role, and prospective students should be aware at least of the powerful influence exerted by the government on the profession and the practitioner. In fact, it might be said that one of the distinguishing marks of the many committed clinical laboratory professionals is their active involvement in the governance process, at the local, state, or federal level, or any combination. Knowing government's enormous influence on the profession, laboratory practitioners in leadership positions tend to assume responsibility for the appropriateness of the laws and regulations that affect their profession. They participate and encourage their colleagues to participate as private citizens in the process of electing and communicating with lawmakers and other public officials. They also exercise this responsibility by participating and encouraging their colleagues to participate in one of the national associations representing the profession. Such groups provide mechanisms by which pending federal and state legislative and regulatory developments are monitored and assessed. They also are the source of many new legislative and regulatory proposals. And they provide a means through which the views of their members can be expressed effectively to lawmakers and other government officials.

CONCLUSION

Competition, law and regulation, health care cost containment, and new scientific and technical developments are issues vital to the clinical laboratory practitioner. Those considering this field should be aware that it is an exciting time to be a clinical laboratory professional.

APPENDIX A

KEY WORDS AND DEFINITIONS

The authors acknowledge the contribution of *Webster's Medical Desk Dictionary*, 1986 edition, and *Saunders Dictionary and Encyclopedia of Laboratory Medicine and Technology*, 1984 edition, for selected terms included in this glossary.

Accreditation: The process by which an agency or organization evaluates and recognizes a program of study or an institution as meeting predetermined qualifications or standards. Example: The Committee on Allied Health Education and Accreditation (CAHEA) accredits various education programs in the clinical laboratory sciences.

Acquired immunodeficiency syndrome (AIDS): A syndrome characterized by a deficiency in the immune system and associated with malignancy and infection. The cause has been identified as HIV, a retrovirus.

Ambulatory care: Diagnostic and treatment services for patients who are capable of walking and able to come and go at will, and not confined to a bed or an institution.

Analyte: In clinical chemistry, the component being measured by an analysis, for example, potassium in a serum potassium assay.

Anatomic pathology: The subspecialty of pathology that deals with the diagnosis of disease from the gross and microscopic examination of tissues and cells removed from patients during surgery, by biopsy, or during postmortem (autopsy) examination.

Anemia: A general condition resulting from a reduction below normal of either the quantity of hemoglobin or number of red blood cells in blood. Symptoms include pallor, fatigue, decreased activity.

Antibody: Any of various proteins (immunoglobulins) in the blood that are generated in reaction to foreign substances to neutralize them. Antibodies produce immunity against cells, microorganisms, or their toxins.

Antigen: A substance, usually a protein, that when introduced into the body stimulates the production of an immune response.

Atherosclerosis: A progressive disease of the vessels characterized by hardening and thickening of the arteries, and usually caused by deposits of cholesterol.

Autoimmunity: A state in which an immune response is generated against components of the individual's own body. Examples of autoimmune diseases include rheumatoid arthritis, thyroiditis, Addison's disease, and multiple sclerosis.

Bacteriology: The science and study of bacteria; specifically, in medicine with those causing disease. Bacteria are usually 1 mm x 4 mm and shaped in rod, spherical, or spiral forms.

Bile: A liquid produced by the liver, usually golden brown, and important in digestion, especially of fats.

Biogenetics: The science of generating new living organisms from other living organisms. "Bioengineering" is sometimes used as a synonym.

Biohazard: An infectious agent that presents a risk to the well-being of humans or animals. Examples of biohazards include viruses, bacteria, fungi, and parasites.

Blood bank: A laboratory area responsible for the preparation of blood, plasma and blood components, and the accurate typing and crossmatching of these products for safe transfusion.

Blood groups: Red cell expression of various antigens; common blood groups tested for include the ABO and Rh systems.

Calibrate: To standardize (usually a measuring instrument such as one used in chemistry) and correct any deviation.

"Call" (to take call or be on call): The expression that denotes a person being ready to respond. A person on call may be at home or near a health care facility, but must be available to return to the institution to work as needed.

Carcinoma: A malignant tumor.

Cerebrospinal fluid (CSF): The clear, colorless fluid that fills spaces within and around the central nervous system (CNS). In an adult, about 500 ml of CSF is formed from plasma each day.

Certification: The process by which a nongovernmental agency or association grants recognition to an individual who has met certain predetermined qualifications specified by that agency as prerequisites for competent practice. Example: The National Certification Agency for Medical Laboratory Personnel certifies individuals for practice through qualifying examinations. Other certifying agencies include the Board of Registry of the American Society of Clinical Pathologists, and the American Medical Technologists. In contrast to licensure, certification is voluntary.

Chemistry (clinical):   The science that deals with the analysis of blood and body fluids to determine their chemical composition.

Chemotherapy: The treatment of disease by chemical agents; especially the treatment of cancer through the use of drugs.

Clinical laboratory: A facility in which analyses are performed on materials derived from the human body for the purpose of providing information for the diagnosis, prevention, or treatment of any disease or impairment; or for assessing, monitoring, and encouraging good health; or for monitoring and assessing the effectiveness of treatment protocols.

Clinical laboratory scientist: Following the certification terminology of the National Certification Agency for Medical Laboratory Personnel, a clinical laboratory scientist is a person who is certified by NCA as a generalist practitioner of clinical laboratory science who uses the credential CLS(NCA). In the certification terminology of the Board of Registry, a clinical laboratory scientist is a certified medical technologist who uses the credential MT(ASCP).

Coagulation (hemostasis):   The study of blood clotting, involving at least twelve factors whose absence, diminution, or excess may lead to abnormalities in clotting; or the process by which platelets and clotting factors interact resulting in the formation of a blood clot.

Compatibility testing: Various procedures used (for example, blood typing and cross-matching) to determine the compatibility of a donor's blood with that of a recipient.

Culture: The growth of microorganisms or living tissue cells in special laboratory media capable of supporting their growth. Most bacteriologic specimens are "cultured" to determine whether bacteria are present and can be identified.

Cytogenetics: The study of the structure and abnormalities of chromosomes. Chromosomal abnormalities are important because of their involvement in birth defects, mental retardation, and spontaneous abortion.

Cytology: The study of cells—their origin, structure, function, and pathology. Clinical cytology is also referred to as cytopathology.

Diabetes: A general term used to characterize excessive production and excretion of urine. Most cases of diabetes are due to insufficient secretion of insulin, causing very high glucose levels, which the body tries to clear through excessive urine output.

Down's syndrome: A group of physical, mental, and functional abnormalities that result from the presence of three (not two) chromosomes at position 21.

Embolism: The sudden blocking of an artery resulting in decreased blood flow. The obstructing agent is usually a clot.

Endocrinology: The study of the system of cells that produce hormones, as well as the management of patients suffering from endocrine disorders, such as diabetes, thyroiditis, or hyperparathyroidism.

Enzyme: Any of complex proteins produced by living organisms and that function as biochemical catalysts.

Forensic medicine: The application of medical science to questions of law, usually concerning the determination of the cause of death in a criminal investigation.

Gram stain: The standard staining procedure for visualizing and categorizing bacteria; usually classified as gram positive (purple) and gram negative (pink).

Hematology: The branch of biology that deals with blood cells and the blood forming organs.

Hemolysis: The release of hemoglobin from within red blood cells.

Hemophilia: A general disorder of blood clotting evidenced by prolonged oozing of blood following minor trauma or surgery.

Hepatitis: Inflammation of the liver that can be caused by viruses, bacteria, fungi, parasites, drugs, or toxins.

Histology: The microscopic study of the structure of cells and tissues. Histology usually includes the techniques of dehydrating, clearing, embedding, and staining tissue sections.

Immunology: The study of the factors involved in the response of an organism to a challenge by a foreign antigen. Immunology involves the study of both normal and abnormal immune function. Abnormal immune functions include hypersensitivity (for example, allergies), autoimmune diseases, and immunodeficiency states.

In vitro: Occurring in an artificial environment outside of the living organism. Example: in a test tube. The majority of laboratory tests are performed "in vitro."

In vivo: Occurring within a living organism.

Independent laboratory: A clinical laboratory that is independent physically and administratively from a hospital, or physician's office, or group practice.

Infectious mononucleosis: A disease caused by the Epstein Barr virus and characterized by fever, fatigue, and atypical lymphocytes in the blood. It is most frequently a disease of young adulthood and usually self-limiting.

Inpatient: A person who is hospitalized.

Iron deficiency anemia: An anemia characterized by low hemoglobin values and small, pale red cells. It is usually associated with dietary deficiency of iron, or chronic blood loss.

Leukemia: A progressive, malignant disease of the blood-forming organs characterized by abnormal kinds and numbers of white blood cells.

Leukocytes (white blood cells): The body's primary defense against infection. They consist of granulocytes (neutrophils, eosinophils, and basophils), lymphocytes, and monocytes.

Licensure: The process by which an agency of government grants permission to persons who meet predetermined qualifications to engage in a given occupation or use a particular title, or grants permission to institutions to perform specified functions. Examples: at the time of publication, California, Florida, Georgia, Hawaii, Nevada, North Dakota, Tennessee, Washington, West Virginia, and New York City required licensure of laboratory practitioners.

Microbiology: A branch of biology dealing with microscopic forms of life, including bacteria, fungi, viruses, rickettsiae, and protozoa.

Monoclonal antibody: An immunochemically identical antibody produced by a simple clone of cells. Monoclonal antibodies are often used to identify cancer cells.

Mycology: The science and study of fungi, including microorganisms such as yeasts or molds.

Myocardial infarct (MI): Heart attack resulting from the death of heart tissue. Most MIs are a result of atherosclerosis of the coronary arteries.

Nosocomial infection: A hospital-acquired infection.

Nuclear medicine: The medical specialty concerned with the use of radioisotopes for in vivo and in vitro tests for the diagnosis and treatment of disease.

Oncology: The study of cancer and cancer-related diseases.

Outpatient: A person who comes to a hosptial, clinic, or other health facility for tests or treatment, but is not admitted to the institution.

Parasitology: The science and study of parasites, organisms that "live off other organisms." An example includes the malaria parasite.

Pathology: The study of the nature of diseases and of the structural and functional changes produced by them.

Physiology: The biological science that deals with how living organisms function, and of the physical and chemical factors and processes involved.

Plasma: A clear, yellowish fluid that accounts for fifty-five percent of the blood volume. It is comprised of ninety-two percent water, seven percent protein and one percent salts, gases, hormones, etc.

Prognosis: The expected outcome, or prospects of recovery from a disease.

Quality control: The process of checking the accuracy and precision of laboratory results and instrument function.

Radioimmunoassay: A laboratory procedure that measures minute quantities of a variety of substances such as hormones, vitamins, drugs, and enzymes by combining the sensitivity of a radioisotope measurement with the specificity of an antibody.

Renal: Related to the kidney.

Reye's syndrome: An acute disease in children thought to be a result of a viral infection and resulting in brain inflammation and liver disease. An association with aspirin ingestion has been made.

Rickettsia: A group of microorganisms that are intermediate between viruses and bacteria. They cause many diseases, for example, typhus, and are usually transmitted by fleas, ticks, or mites.

Septicemia: A systemic infection caused by pathogenic microorganisms, such as bacteria, and characterized by chills and fever. If untreated, septicemia can lead to serious consequences including death.

Serology: The study of antigen-antibody reactions, using a variety of immunologic methods.

Serum: Plasma from which fibrinogen has been removed. (The fluid remaining after a blood clot has formed.)

Sickle cell anemia: An anemia characterized by red cells taking on a sickle shape; these cells are very fragile and have a shortened survival.

Specimen: A preparation of a tissue, organ, or organism for the study of its structure. In laboratories, specimens may include blood, serum, spinal fluid, urine, and other body products.

Staff (or "bench") technologist: A laboratory professional who performs laboratory procedures "at the bench." Staff technologists comprise the major percentage of laboratory professionals. Often, they rotate among laboratory areas. They are responsible for organizing, performing, and reporting the results of their analyses. Most entry-level laboratory positions are at the staff level.

Therapeutic drug monitoring (TDM): A variety of chemistry analyses used to establish whether intended drugs, for example, lithium, used to treat a manic-depressive disorder, are both therapeutically adequate and nontoxic to the user.

Thrombocytopenia: A decrease in the number of blood platelets.

Tissue typing: A means of determining similarities and variations among histocompatability antigens on lymphocytes, so as to optimally match a donor organ (for example, kidney or heart) with a recipient.

Toxic shock syndrome: A disease strongly linked to the bacterium *Staphylococcus aureas;* symptoms include fever, sunburn-like rash, decreased blood pressure. There is an association of toxic shock syndrome with the use of tampons.

Toxicology: The science of poisons: their effects, metabolism, and mechanisms of action. Many clinical chemistry laboratories include a toxicology section to detect and quantitate drugs and poisons.

Tumor (neoplasm): An abnormal mass of cells usually showing uncontrolled and progressive growth.

Urinalysis: The study of urine to identify chemicals and cellular materials present in both normal and abnormal urine.

Virology: The science and study of viruses, minute organisms not visible using an ordinary microscope.

ACRONYMS OF ORGANIZATIONS AND AGENCIES

AAB	American Association of Bioanalysts
AABB	American Association of Blood Banks
AACC	American Association for Clinical Chemistry
ABCP	American Board of Cardiovascular Perfusion
AHA	American Hospital Association
AMA	American Medical Association
AmSECT	American Society of Extra-Corporeal Technology
AMT	American Medical Technologists
ASAHP	American Society of Allied Health Professions
ASC	American Society of Cytology
ASCP	American Society of Clinical Pathologists
ASET	American Society of Electroencephalographic Technologists
ASM	American Society for Microbiology
ASMT	American Society for Medical Technology
ASUTS	American Society of Ultrasound Technical Specialists
BHPr	Bureau of Health Professions
CAP	College of American Pathologists
CDC	Centers for Disease Control
CLIA	Clinical Laboratory Improvement Act (1967, 1988)
CME (AMA)	Council on Medical Education of the American Medical Association
COPA	Council on Postsecondary Accreditation
DHHS	Department of Health and Human Services; formerly Health, Education, and Welfare
ED	U.S. Department of Education

EEOC	Equal Employment Opportunity Commission
EPA	Environmental Protection Agency
FDA	Food and Drug Administration
FMCS	Federal Mediation and Conciliation Service
FTC	Federal Trade Commission
HCFA	Health Care Financing Administration
HMO	Health Maintenance Organization
HRA	Health Resources Administration
HSA	Health Services Administration
JCAHO	Joint Commission on Accreditation of Healthcare Organizations
NAACLS	National Accrediting Agency for Clinical Laboratory Sciences
NCAMLP	National Certification Agency for Medical Laboratory Personnel
NCCLS	National Committee for Clinical Laboratory Standards
NCI	National Cancer Institute
NIH	National Institutes of Health
NIOSH	National Institute of Occupational Safety and Health
NLRB	National Labor Relations Board
NRC	Nuclear Regulatory Commission
NSH	National Society for Histotechnology
OFCC	Office of Federal Contract Compliance
OHD	Office of Human Development
OSHA	Occupational Safety and Health Administration
PHS	Public Health Service
PSRO	Professional Standards Review Organization
SDMS	Society of Diagnostic Medical Sonographers
SNM	Society of Nuclear Medicine
SNM-TS	Society of Nuclear Medicine-Technologist Section
SSA	Social Security Administration
USA	United States Army
USAF	United States Air Force
USN	United States Navy
USOE	United States Office of Education
USPHS	United States Public Health Services
VA	Department of Veterans Affairs; formerly Veterans Administration

ORGANIZATIONS AND ADDRESSES

Accrediting Organizations for Laboratory Education Programs

Accrediting Bureau of Health
  Education Schools
Oak Manor Office
29089 U.S. 20 West
Elkhart, IN 46514
(219) 293-0124

Committee on Allied Health
  Education and Accreditation
  (CAHEA)
535 North Dearborn Street
Chicago, IL 60610
(312) 751-6272

National Accrediting Agency for
  Clinical Laboratory Sciences
  (NAACLS)
Suite 608
547 West Jackson Boulevard
Chicago, IL 60606-5717
(312) 461-0333

Certifying Agencies for Graduates of Laboratory Education Programs

American Medical Technologists
  (AMT)
AMT Building
710 Higgins Road
Park Ridge, IL 60068
(312) 823-5169

Board of Registry of American
  Society of Clinical Pathologists
P.O. Box 12270
Chicago, IL 60612
(312) 738-1336

National Certification Agency for
  Medical Laboratory Personnel
  (NCA)
2021 L Street NW, Suite 400
Washington, DC 20036
(202) 857-1023

Professional Organizations of Interest for Laboratory Personnel

American Association of Bioanalysts
(AAB)
Suite 918, 818 Olive Street
St. Louis, MO 63101
(314) 241-1445

American Association of Blood
Banks (AABB)
Suite 600, 1117 North 19th Street
Arlington, VA 22209
(703) 528-8200

American Association for Clinical
Chemistry (AACC)
2029 K Street, NW, 7th Floor
Washington, DC 20006
(202) 875-0717

American Association of
Immunologists (AAI)
9650 Rockville Pike
Bethesda, MD 20814
(301) 530-7178

American Association of
Pathologists' Assistants (AAPA)
7389 Crawford Drive
Gilroy, CA 95020
(209) 225-3000 X1505

American Hospital Association
(AHA)
840 North Lake Shore Drive
Chicago, IL 60611
(312) 280-6000

American Medical
Electroencephalographic
Association
850 Elm Grove Road
Elm Grove, WI 53122
(414) 784-3646

American Society of Clinical
Pathologists
2100 West Harrison Street
Chicago, IL 60612
(312) 738-1336

American Society of Cytology (ASC)
1015 Chestnut Street, Suite 1518
Philadelphia, PA 19107
(215) 922-3880

American Society of Hematology
(ASH)
6900 Grove Road
Thoroughfare, NJ 08086
(609) 845-0003

American Society for Medical
Technology (ASMT)
2021 L Street NW, Suite 400
Washington, DC 20036
(202) 785-3311

American Society for Microbiology
1913 I Street NW
Washington, DC 20006
(202) 833-9680

Canadian Society of Laboratory
Technologists (CSLT)
P.O. Box 2830 Station A
Hamilton, Ont. L8N 3N5
(416) 538-8642

Clinical Laboratory Management
   Association (CLMA)
193-195 West Lancaster Avenue
Paoli, PA 19301
(215) 647-8970

International Association of Medical
   Laboratory Technologists
   (IAMLT)
1 Drayton Gardens
Winchmore Hill, London N21 2 NT
United Kingdom

International Society for Clinical
   Laboratory Technology (ISCLT)
818 Olive Street, Suite 918
St. Louis, MO 63101
(314) 241-1445

National Society for Histotechnology
5900 Princess Garden Parkway,
   Suite 805
Lanham, MD 20706
(301) 577-4907

Society of Nuclear Medicine (SNM)
316 Madison Avenue
New York, NY 10016
(212) 889-0717

ACCREDITED CLINICAL LABORATORY SCIENCE/MEDICAL TECHNOLOGY PROGRAMS

Following are the professional medical technology programs at the baccalaureate level that are accredited by the Committee on Allied Health Education and Accreditation (CAHEA). In some instances, the accredited program involves only the fourth year and is located at a hospital. Students are advised to write the program director of these hospitals to obtain the names and addresses of colleges and universities that offer prerequisite courses. In other instances, the accredited program is listed as the university or college which is responsible for both the preprofessional and professional program. In this case, all course work may be taken at one institution.

Alabama

Baptist Medical Centers-Montclair
Medical Technologist Program
800 Montclair Road
Birmingham, AL 35213

University of Alabama at Birmingham
School/Health Related Professions
Medical Technologist Program
University Station
Birmingham, AL 35294

University of South Alabama
Medical Technologist Program
494 Cancer Center/Clinical
Building
Mobile, AL 36688-0001

Auburn University at Montgomery
School of Science/Department of
Biology
Medical Technologist Program
Montgomery, AL 36193

Baptist Medical Center
Medical Technologist Program
2105 East South Boulevard
Montgomery, AL 36198

St. Margaret's Hospital
Medical Technologist Program
301 South Ripley Street, Drawer
311
Montgomery, AL 36195

Tuskegee University
Medical Technologist Program
Basil O'Connor Hall
Tuskegee, AL 36088

Arizona

Arizona State University
Clinical Lab Sciences
Medical Technologist Program
Department Botany/Microbiology
Tempe, AZ 85287

University Medical Center
Medical Technologist Program
1435 North Fremont
Tucson, AZ 85719

Arkansas

Arkansas College
Medical Technologist Program
2300 Highland Road
Batesville, AR 72501

Baptist Medical System
Medical Technologist Program
9601 Interstate 630, Exit 7
Little Rock, AR 72205-7299

University of Arkansas for Medical
Sciences
Medical Technologist Program
4301 West Markham Slot 597
Little Rock, AR 72205

Arkansas State University
Medical Technologist Program
P.O. Box 69
State University, AR 72467

California

California State College
Medical Technologist Program
9001 Stockdale Highway
Bakersfield, CA 93309

California State University
Medical Technologist Program
1000 East Victoria Street
Carson, CA 90747

Fresno Community Hospital and
Medical Center
Medical Technologist Program
P.O. Box 1232
Fresno, CA 93715

Valley Children's Hospital
Medical Technologist Program
3151 North Milbrook Avenue
Fresno, CA 93703

Centinela Hospital Medical Center
Medical Technologist Program
555 East Hardy Street
P.O. Box 720
Inglewood, CA 90301

Scripps Clinic and Research
Foundation
Medical Technologist Program
10666 North Torrey Pines Road
211C
La Jolla, CA 92037

Scripps Memorial Hospital
Medical Technologist Program
9888 Genesee Avenue
La Jolla, CA 92037

Grossmont District Hospital
Laboratory
Medical Technologist Program
5555 Grossmont Center Drive
La Mesa, CA 92042

Loma Linda University
Medical Technologist Program
Office of the Dean
Loma Linda, CA 92350

St. Mary Medical Center Bauer
Hospital
Medical Technologist Program
1050 Linden Avenue
Long Beach, CA 90813

VA Medical Center
Medical Technologist Program
5901 East 7th Street
Long Beach, CA 90822

Cedars Sinai Medical Center
Medical Technologists Program
8700 Beverly Boulevard
Los Angeles, CA 90048

Children's Hospital of Los Angeles
Medical Technologist Program
4650 Sunset Boulevard
Los Angeles, CA 90027

King/Drew Medical Center
Medical Technologist Program
12021 South Wilmington Avenue
Los Angeles, CA 90059

Los Angeles County-USC Medical
Center
Medical Technologist Program
12021 North State Street
Los Angeles, CA 90033

UCLA Center for Health Sciences
Medical Technologist Program
10833 Le Conte Avenue
Los Angeles, CA 90024-1713

VA Wadsworth Medical Center
Medical Technologist Program
Wilshire and Sawtelle Boulevards
Los Angeles, CA 90073

VA Medical Center
Medical Technologist Program
150 Muir Road
Martinez, CA 94553

El Camino Hospital
Medical Technologist Program
2500 Grant Road
Mountain View, CA 94040

St. Joseph Hospital
Medical Technologist Program
1100 Stewart Drive, P.O. Box 5600
Orange, CA 92268

Huntington Memorial Hospital
Medical Technologist Program
100 Congress Street
Pasadena, CA 91105

Eisenhower Medical Center
Medical Technologist Program
39000 Bob Hope Drive
Rancho Mirage, CA 92270

University of California Davis
Medical Center
Medical Technologist Program
2315 Stockton Boulevard
Sacramento, CA 95817

San Bernardino County Medical
Center
Medical Technologist Program
780 East Gilbert Street
San Bernardino, CA 92404

Sharp Memorial Hospital
Medical Technologist Program
7901 Frost Street
San Diego, CA 92123

Children's Hospital of San Francisco
Medical Technologist Program
3700 California Street
San Francisco, CA 94118

San Francisco State University
Medical Technologist Program
Center for Advanced Medical
Technology
San Francisco, CA 94132

San Jose Medical Center
Medical Technologist Program
675 East Santa Clara Street
San Jose, CA 95112

Santa Clara Valley Medical Center
Medical Technologist Program
751 South Bascom Avenue
San Jose, CA 95128

Santa Barbara Cottage Hospital
Medical Technologist Program
P.O. Box 689, Pueblo at Bath
Streets
Santa Barbara, CA 93102

St. John's Hospital and Health Center
Medical Technologist Program
1328 Twenty-Second Street
Santa Monica, CA 90404

Sepulveda VA Medical Center
Medical Technologist Program
16111 Plummer Street
Sepulveda, CA 91343

LA County Harbor UCLA Medical
Center
Medical Technologist Program
1000 West Carson Street
Torrance, CA 90509

Colorado

Memorial Hospital
Medical Technologist Program
1400 East Boulder Street
Colorado Springs, CO 80909

Penrose Hospitals
Medical Technologist Program
2215 Cascade Avenue, P.O. 7021
Colorado Springs, CO 80933

Presbyterian/St. Luke Center for
Health Science Education
Medical Technologist Program
1719 East 19th Avenue
Denver, CO 80218

University of Colorado Health
   Science Center
Medical Technologist Program
4200 East 9th Avenue, B-173
Denver, CO 80262

North Colorado Medical Center
Medical Technologist Program
1801 16th Street
Greeley, CO 80631

Parkview Episcopal Medical Center
Medical Technologist Program
400 West 16th Street
Pueblo, CO 81003

Connecticut

Bridgeport Hospital
Medical Technologist Program
267 Grant Street
Bridgeport, CT 06602

St. Vincent's Medical Center
Medical Technologist Program
2800 Main Street
Bridgeport, CT 06606

Danbury Hospital
Medical Technologist Program
24 Hospital Avenue
Danbury, CT 06810

Quinnipiac College
Medical Technologist Program
Mt. Carmel Avenue
Hamden, CT 06518

Hartford Hospital
Medical Technologist Program
80 Seymour Street
Hartford, CT 06115

St. Joseph Medical Center
Medical Technologist Program
128 Strawberry Hill Avenue
P.O. Box 1222
Stamford, CT 06904

St. Mary's Hospital
Medical Technologist Program
56 Franklin Street
Waterbury, CT 06702

Waterbury Hospital Health Center
Medical Technologist Program
64 Robbins Street
Waterbury, CT 06721

University of Hartford
Medical Technologist Program
Dana Hall, Room 232
200 Bloomfield Avenue
West Hartford, CT 06117-1599

Delaware

Wesley College
Medical Technologist Program
College Square
Dover, DE 19901

University of Delaware
Medical Technologist Program
117 Wolf Hall
Newark, DE 19716

District of Columbia

Catholic University of America
Medical Technologist Program
620 Michigan Avenue NE
Washington, DC 20064

George Washington University
   Medical Center
   Medical Technologist Program
   2300 Eye Street NW
   Washington, DC 20037

Howard University
   Medical Technologist Program
   6th and Bryant Street NW, C/AHS
   Washington, DC 20059

Walter Reed Army Medical Center
   Clinical Lab Officer Course
   6825 16th Street NW, Room 2B72
   Washington, DC 20037-5001

Washington Hospital Center
   Medical Technologist Program
   110 Irving Street NW
   Washington, DC 20010

Florida

Florida Atlantic University
   Medical Technologist Program
   NE 20th Street
   Boca Raton, FL 33431

Bethune-Cookman College
   Medical Technologist Program
   640 Second Avenue
   Daytona Beach, FL 32015

University of Florida
   Health Science Center
   Medical Technologist Program
   Health Science Center, Box J-194
   Gainesville, FL 32610

Baptist Medical Center
   Medical Technologist Program
   800 Prudential Drive
   Jacksonville, FL 32207

St. Vincent's Medical Center
   Medical Technologist Program
   1800 Barrs Street, P.O. Box 2982
   Jacksonville, FL 32203

University Hospital of Jacksonville
   Medical Technologist Program
   655 West 8th Street
   Jacksonville, FL 32209

Florida International University
   Medical Technologist Program
   University Park Campus
   Miami, FL 33199

Mt. Sinai Medical Center
   Medical Technologist Program
   4300 Alton Road
   Miami Beach, FL 33140

Florida Hospital
   Medical Technologist Program
   601 East Rollins
   Orlando, FL 32803

University of Central Florida
   Medical Technologist Program
   P.O. Box 25000
   Orlando, FL 32816

University of West Florida
   Department of Biology
   Medical Technologist Program
   11000 University Parkway
   Pensacola, FL 32514-5751

Bayfront Medical Center
   Medical Technologist Program
   701 Sixth Street South
   St. Petersburg, FL 33701

Tallahassee Memorial Regional
   Medical Center
Medical Technologist Program
Magnolia and Miccousukee Roads
Tallahassee, FL 32308

Tampa General Hospital
Medical Technologist Program
P.O. Box 1289
Tampa, FL 33601

Georgia

Crawford Long Hospital of Emory
   University
Medical Technologist Program
550 Peachtree Street NE
Atlanta, GA 30365

Emory University Hospital
Medical Technologist Program
1364 Clifton Road NE
Atlanta, GA 30322

Georgia Baptist Medical Center
Medical Technologist Program
300 Boulevard NE
Atlanta, GA 30312

Georgia State University
Medical Technologist Program
University Plaza
Atlanta, GA 30303-3090

Grady Memorial Hospital
Medical Technologist Program
80 Butler Street SE
Atlanta, GA 30335-3801

Medical College of Georgia
Medical Technologist Program
August, GA 30912-1650

Columbus College
Medical Technologist Program
Algonquin Drive
Columbus, GA 31993-2399

Armstrong State College
Medical Technologist Program
11935 Abercorn Street
Savannah, GA 31406

Hawaii

St. Francis Hospital
Medical Technologist Program
2230 Liliha Street
Honolulu, HI 96817

University of Hawaii at Manoa
Medical Technologist Program
2538 The Mall, Snyder 407
Honolulu, HI 96822

Idaho

St. Alphonsus Regional Medical
   Center
Medical Technologist Program
1055 North Curtis Road
Boise, ID 83706

Illinois

St. Elizabeth Hospital
Medical Technologist Program
211 South Third Street
Belleville, IL 62222

Louis A. Weiss Memorial Hospital
Medical Technologist Program
4646 North Marine Drive
Chicago, IL 60640

Rush Presbyterian St. Luke's Medical
Center
Medical Technologist Program
1753 West Congress Parkway
Chicago, IL 60612

St. Joseph Hospital
Medical Technologist Program
2900 North Lake Shore Drive
Chicago, IL 60657

University of Illinois at Chicago
Medical Technologist Program
808 South Wood Street, 690 CME
Chicago, IL 60612

United Samaritans Medical Center
Medical Technologist Program
812 North Logan Avenue
Danville, IL 61832

Decatur Memorial Hospital
Medical Technology Program
2300 North Edward Street
Decatur, IL 62526

National College of Education
Medical Technologist Program
2840 Sheridan Road
Evanston, IL 60201

Edward Hines Jr., VA Hospital
Medical Technologist Program-113
Fifth Avenue and Roosevelt Road
Hines, IL 60141

Hinsdale Hospital
Medical Technologist Program
120 North Oak Street
Hinsdale, IL 60521

Foster G. McGaw Hospital of Loyola
University
Medical Technologist Program
2160 South First Avenue
Maywood, IL 60153

University of Health Science/Chicago
Medical School
Medical Technologist Program
3333 Greenbay Road
North Chicago, IL 60064

Christ Hospital
Medical Technologist Program
4440 West 95th Street
Oak Lawn, IL 60453

Methodist Medical Center of Illinois
Medical Technologist Program
221 Northeast Glen Oak Avenue
Peoria, IL 61636

St. Francis Medical Center
Medical Technologist Program
530 Northeast Glen Oak Avenue
Peoria, IL 61637

Rockford Memorial Hospital
Medical Technologist Program
2400 North Rockton Avenue
Rockford, IL 61103

St. Anthony Medical Center
Medical Technologist Program
5666 East State Street
Rockford, IL 61108

Swedish American Hospital
Medical Technologist Program
1400 Charles Street
Rockford, IL 61104

Sangamon State University
Medical Technologist Program
Shepherd Road
Springfield, IL 62794

St. John's Hospital
Medical Technologist Program
800 East Carpenter
Springfield, IL 62769

Governors State University
Medical Technology Program
Route 54 and Stuenkel Road
University Park, IL 60466

Indiana

St. Francis Hospital Center
Medical Technologist Program
1600 Albany Street
Beech Grove, IN 46107

St. Mary's Medical Center
Medical Technologist Program
3700 Washington Avenue
Evansville, IN 47750

Lutheran Hospital of Indiana
Medical Technologist Program
3024 Fairfield Avenue
Fort Wayne, IN 46807

Parkview Memorial Hospital
Medical Technologist Program
2200 Randallia
Fort Wayne, IN 46805

St. Joseph Medical Center
Medical Technologist Program
700 Broadway
Fort Wayne, IN 46802

St. Margaret Hospital and Health
Centers
Medical Technologist Program
5454 Hohman Avenue
Hammond, IN 46320

St. Mary Medical Center
Medical Technologist Program
1500 South Lake Park Avenue
Hobart, IN 46342

Indiana University School of Medicine
Medical Technologist Program
Fesler Hall Room 416, 1120 South
Drive
Indianapolis, IN 46223

Methodist Hospital of Indiana
Medical Technologist Program
1701 North Senate Boulevard,
P.O. 1367
Indianapolis, IN 46206

St. Vincent Hospital and Health Care
Center
Medical Technologist Program
2001 West 86th Street, Box 40970
Indianapolis, IN 46240-0970

St. Joseph Hospital and Health Center
Medical Technologist Program
1907 West Sycamore Street
Kokomo, IN 46901

Ball Memorial Hospital
Medical Technologist Program
2401 University Avenue
Muncie, IN 47303

Indiana State University
Medical Technologist Program
217 North 6th Street
Terre Haute, IN 47809

Good Samaritan Hospital
Medical Technologist Program
520 South Seventh Street
Vincennes, IN 47591

Iowa

St. Lukes Hospital
Medical Technologist Program
1026 "A" Avenue NE
Cedar Rapids, IA 52402

Iowa Methodist Medical Center
Medical Technologist Program
1200 Pleasant Street
Des Moines, IA 50309

Mercy Hospital Medical Center
Medical Technologist Program
Mercy Court, 921 6th Avenue
Des Moines, IA 50314

University of Iowa
U of Iowa Hospitals and Clinics
Pathology
Medical Technologist Program
150A Medical Laboratories
Iowa City, IA 52242

Marian Health Center
Medical Technologist Program
801 5th Street
Sioux City, IA 51101

St. Luke's Medical Center
Medical Technologist Program
2720 Stone Park Boulevard
Sioux City, IA 51104

Consolidated Regional Laboratories
Medical Technologist Program
c/o Covenant Medical Center
3421 West 9th Street
Waterloo, IA 50702

Kansas

Providence St. Margaret Health Center
Medical Technologist Program
8929 Parallel Parkway
Kansas City, KS 66112

University of Kansas Medical Center
Medical Technologist Program
39th Street and Rainbow Boulevard
Kansas City, KS 66103

Topeka School of Medical Technology
Medical Technologist Program
1505 West 8th Street
Topeka, KS 66606

Wichita State University
Department of Clinical Sciences
Medical Technologist Program
P.O. Box 43
Wichita, KS 67208

Kentucky

St. Elizabeth Medical Center
Medical Technologist Program
One Medical Village Drive
Edgewood, KY 41017

University of Kentucky
Medical Technologist Program
122 Medical Center Annex 2
Lexington, KY 40536

University of Louisville
Medical Technologist Program
Health Sciences Center
Louisville, KY 40292

Owensboro Daviess County Hospital
Medical Technologist Program
12th and Triplett Streets, P.O. Box
2799
Owensboro, KY 42302

Lourdes Hospital
Medical Technologist Program
1530 Lone Oak Road
Paducah, KY 42001

Methodist Hospital of Kentucky
911 South ByPass
Pikeville, KY 41505

Eastern Kentucky University
Medical Technologist Program
Wallace 111
Richmond, KY 40475

Louisiana

Rapides General Hospital
Medical Technologist Program
211 Fourth Street, Box 30101
Alexandria, LA 71301

Earl K. Long Memorial Hospital
Medical Technologist Program
5825 Airline Highway
Baton Rouge, LA 70805

Our Lady of the Lake Regional
Medical Center
Medical Technologist Program
5000 Hennessy Boulevard
Baton Rouge, LA 70805

University Medical Center
Medical Technologist Program
2390 West Congress, P.O. Box
4016-C
Lafayette, LA 70502

Lake Charles Memorial Hospital
School of Medical Technology
Medical Technologist Program
1701 Oak Park Boulevard
Lake Charles, LA 70601

St. Patrick Hospital
Medical Technologist Program
524 South Ryan Street
P.O. Box 3401
Lake Charles, LA 70602-3401

St. Francis Medical Center
309 Jackson Street
Monroe, LA 71201

Alton Ochsner Medical Foundation
1516 Jefferson Highway
New Orleans, LA 70121

Charity Hospital of Louisiana-New
Orleans
Medical Technologist Program
1532 Tulane Avenue
New Orleans, LA 70140

Louisiana State University Medical
Center
Medical Technologist Program
1900 Gravier Street
New Orleans, LA 70112

Touro Infirmary School of Medical
Technology
Medical Technologist Program
1401 Foucher Street
New Orleans, LA 70115

Veterans Administration Medical
Center
Medical Technologist Program
1601 Perdido Street
New Orleans, LA 70146

Overton Brooks VA Medical Center
Medical Technologist Program
510 East Stoner Avenue
Shreveport, LA 71101-4295

Schumpert Medical Center
Medical Technologist Program
P.O. Box 21976
Shreveport, LA 71120-1976

Maine

Eastern Maine Medical Center
Medical Technologist Program
489 State Street
Bangor, ME 04401

Maine Medical Center
Medical Technologist Program
22 Bramhall Street
Portland, ME 04102-3175

Maryland

Mercy Hospital
Medical Technologist Program
301 St. Paul Street
Baltimore, MD 21202

Morgan State University
Medical Technologist Program
Coldspring Lane and Hillen Road
Baltimore, MD 21239

Union Memorial Hospital
Medical Technologist Program
201 East University Parkway
Baltimore, MD 21218

University of Maryland School of
    Medicine
Medical Technologist Program
32 South Green Street
Baltimore, MD 21201

Oscar B. Hunter Memorial Library
Medical Technologist Program
8218 Wisconsin Avenue, Suite 202
Bethesda, MD 20814

Malcolm Grow USAF Medical Center
Medical Technologist Program
Andrews AFB, DC
Camp Springs, MD 20331-5300

Salisbury State College
Medical Technologist Program
Camden Avenue
Salisbury, MD 21801

Columbia Union College
Medical Technologist Program
7600 Flower Avenue
Takoma Park, MD 20912

Massachusetts

New England Deaconess Hospital
Medical Technologist Program
185 Pilgrim/Mssnr Lab G22
Boston, MA 02215

Northeastern University
Medical Technologist Program
360 Huntington Avenue
Boston, MA 02215

Veterans Administration Medical
    Center
Medical Technologist Program
150 South Huntington Avenue
Boston, MA 02130

Cambridge Hospital
Medical Technologist Program
1493 Cambridge Street
Cambridge, MA 02139

Fitchburg State College
Medical Technology Program
Fitchburg, MA 01420

Lawrence General Hospital
Medical Technologist Program
1 General Street
Lawrence, MA 01842

University of Lowell
Medical Technologist Program
Weed Hall 1, University Avenue
Lowell, MA 01854

Newton Wellesley Hospital
Medical Technologist Program
2014 Washington Street
Newton Lower Falls, MA 02162

Southeastern Massachusetts University
Medical Technology Department
Medical Technologist Program
Old Westport Road
North Dartmouth, MA 02747

Berkshire Medical Center
Medical Technologist Program
725 North Street
Pittsfield, MA 01201

Baystate Medical Center
Medical Technologist Program
759 Chestnut Street
Springfield, MA 01199

Mercy Hospital
Medical Technologist Program
271 Carew Street, P.O. Box 9012
Springfield, MA 01102-9012

Michigan

Ferris State University
Medical Technologist Program
VFS 404
Big Rapids, MI 49307

Hutzel Hospital
Medical Technologist Program
4707 Saint Antoine
Detroit, MI 48201

Mercy College of Detroit
Medical Technologist Program
8200 West Outer Drive
Detroit, MI 48219

St. John Hospital
Medical Technologist Program
22101 Moross Road
Detroit, MI 48236

Wayne State University
Medical Technologist Program
233 Shapero Hall
Detroit, MI 48202

Michigan State University
Medical Technologist Program
122 Natural Sciences Building
East Lansing, MI 48824

Hurley Medical Center
Medical Technologist Program
Number One Hurley Plaza
Flint, MI 48502

St. Joseph Hospital
Medical Technologist Program
302 Kensington Avenue
Flint, MI 48502

Garden City Hospital, Osteopathic
Medical Technologist Program
6245 North Inkster Road
Garden City, MI 48135

Butterworth Hospital
Medical Technologist Program
100 Michigan Street NE
Grand Rapids, MI 49503

W. A. Foote Memorial Hospital
Medical Technologist Program
205 North East Avenue
Jackson, MI 49201

Edward W. Sparrow Hospital
Association
Medical Technologist Program
1215 East Michigan, P.O. 30480
Lansig, MI 48909

Northern Michigan Hospitals
Medical Technologist Program
416 Connable Avenue
Petoskey, MI 49770

Pontiac General Hospital
Medical Technologist Program
Department of Laboratories
Pontiac, MI 48053

William Beaumont Hospital
Medical Technologist Program
3601 West 13 Mile Road
Royal Oak, MI 48072

St. Mary's Hospital
Medical Technologist Program
830 South Jefferson Avenue
Saginaw, MI 48601

Providence Hospital
School of Medical Technology
Medical Technologist Program
16001 West Nine Mile Road
Box 2043
Southfield, MI 48037

Munson Medical Center
Medical Technologist Program
1105 Sixth Street
Traverse City, MI 49684

Eastern Michigan University
Medical Technologist Program
327 King Hall
Ypsilanti, MI 48197

Minnesota

College of St. Scholastica
Clinical Laboratory Science
Department
1200 Kenwood Avenue
Duluth, MN 55811

Abbott Northwestern Hospital
Medical Technologist Program
800 East 28th Street at Chicago
Avenue
Minneapolis, MN 55407

Hennepin County Medical Center
Medical Technologist Program
701 Park Avenue South
Minneapolis, MN 55415

University of Minnesota Health
Science Center
Medical Technologist Program
Box 198 UMHC, 420 Delaware
Street, SE
Minneapolis, MN 55455

St. Cloud Hospital
Medical Technologist Program
1406 6th Avenue North
St. Cloud, MN 56301

St. Paul Ramsey Medical Center
Medical Technologist Program
640 Jackson Street
St. Paul, MN 55101

United Hospital
Medical Technologist Program
333 North Smith Avenue
St. Paul, MN 55102

Mississippi

University of Southern Mississippi
Medical Technologist Program
Box 5134 Southern Station
Hattiesburg, MS 39406

William Carey College
Medical Technologist Program
Tuscan Avenue
Hattiesburg, MS 39401

Mississippi Baptist Medical Center
Medical Technologist Program
1225 North State Street
Jackson, MS 39202

University of Mississippi Medical
Center
Medical Technologist Program
2500 North State Street
Jackson, MS 39216

North Mississippi Medical Center
Medical Technologist Program
830 South Gloster
Tupelo, MS 38801

Missouri

St. John's Regional Medical Center
Medical Technologist Program
2727 McClelland Boulevard
Joplin, MO 64804-7170

Avila College
Medical Technologist Program
11901 Wornall Road
Kansas City, MO 64145

Menorah Medical Center
Medical Technologist Program
4949 Rockhill Road
Kansas City, MO 64110

Research Medical Center
Medical Technologist Program
2316 East Meyer Boulevard
Kansas City, MO 64132

St. Luke's Hospital of Kansas City
Medical Technologist Program
4400 Wornall Road
Kansas City, MO 64111

Trinity Lutheran Hospital
Medical Technologist Program
31st and Wyandotte Streets
Kansas City, MO 64108

North Kansas City Hospital
Medical Technologist Program
2800 Hospital Drive
North Kansas City, MO 64116

Cox Medical Centers
Medical Technologist Program
3801 South National Avenue
Springfield, MO 65807

St. John's Regional Health Center
Medical Technologist Program
1235 East Cherokee
Springfield, MO 65804

Jewish Hospital of St. Louis
Medical Technologist Program
216 South Kingshighway Boulevard
St. Louis, MO 63110

St. John's Mercy Medical Center
Medical Technologist Program
615 South New Ballas Road
St. Louis, MO 63141

St. Louis University
Medical Technologist Program
1504 South Grand Boulevard
St. Louis, MO 63104

Montana

St. James Community Hospital
Medical Technologist Program
400 South Clark Street
Butte, MT 59701

Columbus Hospital
Medical Technologist Program
500 15th Avenue South
Great Falls, MT 59403

Nebraska

Bishop Clarkson Memorial Hospital
Medical Technologist Program
44th and Dewey Avenue
Omaha, NE 68105

Nebraska Methodist Hospital
Medical Technologist Program
8303 Dodge Street
Omaha, NE 68114

University of Nebraska Medical
Center
Medical Technologist Program
42nd and Dewey Avenues
Omaha, NE 68105

Nevada

University of Nevada-Reno
Medical Technologist Program
300 MacKay Science Building
Reno, NV 89557

New Hampshire

University of New Hampshire
Medical Technologist Program
Thompson Hall
Durham, NH 03824

Notre Dame College
Medical Technologist Program
2321 Elm Street
Manchester, NH 03104

New Jersey

Cooper Hospital/University Medical
Center
Medical Technologist Program
One Cooper Plaza
Camden, NJ 08103

Monmouth Medical Center
Medical Technologist Program
300 Second Avenue
Long Branch, NJ 07740

Mountainside Hospital
Medical Technologist Program
Bay and Highland Avenues
Montclair, NJ 07042-4898

Morristown Memorial Hospital
Medical Technologist Program
100 Madison Avenue
Morristown, NJ 07960

Jersey Shore Medical Center Fitkin
Hospital
Medical Technologist Program
1945 Corlies Avenue
Neptune, NJ 07753

St. Peter's Medical Center
Medical Technologist Program
254 Easton Avenue
New Brunswick, NJ 08903

University of Medicine and Dentistry
of New Jersey
School of Health Related
Professions
Medical Technologist Program
65 Bergen Street
Newark, NJ 07107-3006

Hospital Center at Orange
Medical Technologist Program
188 South Essex Avenue
Orange, NJ 07051

Bergen Pines County Hospital
Medical Technologist Program
East Ridgewood Avenue
Paramus, NJ 07652

St. Mary's Hospital, Passaic
Medical Technologist Program
211 Pennington Avenue
Passaic, NJ 07055

Barnert Memorial Hospital Center
Medical Technologist Program
680 Broadway
Paterson, NJ 07514

St. Joseph's Hospital Medical Center
Medical Technologist Program
703 Main Street
Paterson, NJ 07503

Valley Hospital
Medical Technologist Program
Linwood and North Van Dien
Avenue
Ridgewood, NJ 07451

Somerset Medical Center
Medical Technologist Program
Rehill Avenue
Somerville, NJ 08876

New Mexico

University of New Mexico School of
Medicine
Medical Technologist Program
Medical Center Building #4
Albuquerque, NM 87131

Memorial General Hospital
Medical Technologist Program
Telshor Boulevard and University
Avenue
Las Cruces, NM 88001

New York

Albany Medical Center Hospital
Medical Technologist Program
New Scotland Avenue
Albany, NY 12208

College of Saint Rose
Medical Technologist Program
432 Western Avenue
Albany, NY 12203

Daemen College
Medical Technologist Program
4380 Main Street
Amherst, NY 14226

Methodist Hospital of Brooklyn
Medical Technologist Program
506 Sixth Street
Brooklyn, NY 11215

Long Island University
CW Post Campus
Medical Technologist Program
Northern Boulevard
Brookvale, NY 11548

Millard Fillmore Hospital
Medical Technologist Program
3 Gates Circle
Buffalo, NY 14209

SUNY Health Science Center at
Buffalo
Medical Technologist Program
462 Grider Street
Buffalo, NY 14215

Women's Christian Association
Hospital
Medical Technologist Program
207 Foote Avenue
Jamestown, NY 14701-7077

Northern Westchester Hospital Center
Medical Technologist Program
East Main Street
Mt. Kisco, NY 10549

Lenox Hill Hospital
Medical Technologist Program
100 East 77th Street
New York, NY 10021-1803

St. Vincent's Hospital and Medical
Center of New York
Medical Technologist Program
153 West 11th Street
New York, NY 10011

Mount Saint Mary College
Medical Technologist Program
330 Powell Avenue
Newburgh, NY 12550

Marist College
Medical Technologist Program
North Road
Poughkeepsie, NY 12601

Rochester General Hospital
Medical Technologist Program
1425 Portland Avenue
Rochester, NY 14621

St. Mary's Hospital
Medical Technologist Program
89 Genesee Street
Rochester, NY 14611

SUNY Health Science Center at Stony
Brook
Medical Technologist Program
Health Science Center-Allied
Health
Stony Brook, NY 11794

SUNY Health Science Center at
Syracuse
Medical Technologist Program
750 Adams Street
Syracuse, NY 13210

Utica College of Syracuse University
Medical Technologist Program
1600 Burrstone Road
Utica, NY 13502

Catholic Medical Center
Medical Technologist Program
88-15 Woodhaven Avenue
Woodhaven, NY 11421

North Carolina

University of North Carolina
Medical Allied Health Professions
Medical Technologist Program
CB# 7120 Medical School Wing E
Chapel Hill, NC 27599-7120

Charlotte Memorial Hospital and
Medical Center
Medical Technologist Program
P.O. Box 32861
Charlotte, NC 28232

Presbyterian Hospital
Medical Technologist Program
200 Hawthorne Lane, Box 33549
Charlotte, NC 28233-3549

Western Carolina University
Medical Technologist Program
134 Moore Hall
Cullowhee, NC 28723

Duke University Medical Center
Medical Technologist Program
Box 2929, Hospital Labs
Durham, NC 27710

Moses H. Cone Memorial Hospital
Medical Technologist Program
1200 North Elm Street
Greensboro, NC 27401

East Carolina University
Medical Technologist Program
School of Allied Health Sciences
Greenville, NC 27858

New Hanover Memorial Hospital
Medical Technologist Program
2131 South 17th Street
P.O. Box 9000
Wilmington, NC 28402-7407

Bowman Gray School of Medicine
Medical Technologist Program
300 South Hawthorne Road
Winston-Salem, NC 27103

Forsyth Memorial Hospital
Medical Technologist Program
3333 Silas Creek Parkway
Winston-Salem, NC 27103

Winston-Salem State University
Medical Technologist Program
P.O. Box 13156
Winston-Salem, NC 27110

North Dakota

St. Alexius Medical Center
Medical Technologist Program
900 East Broadway, Box 1658
Bismarck, ND 58501

St. Luke's Hospital
Medical Technologist Program
737 Broadway, P.O. Box 2067
Fargo, ND 58102

University of North Dakota
Medical Technologist Program
Department of Pathology
Grand Forks, ND 58201

St. Joseph's Hospital
Medical Technologist Program
3rd Street Southeast and Burdick
    Expressway
Minot, ND 58701

Trinity Medical Center
Medical Technologist Program
Main Street and Burdick
Expressway
Minot, ND 58701

Ohio

Children's Hospital Medical Center of
Akron
Coop Medical Technology Program
281 Locust Street
Akron, OH 44308

St. Thomas Medical Center
Medical Technologist Program
444 North Main Street
Akron, OH 44310

University of Cincinnati Medical
Center
Medical Technologist Program
231 Bethesda Avenue
Blue Ash, OH 45267

Bowling Green State University
Medical Technologist Program
504 Life Science Building
Bowling Green, OH 43403

Christ Hospital
Medical Technologist Program
2139 Auburn Avenue
Cincinnati, OH 45219

Providence Hospital
Medical Technologist Program
2446 Kipling Avenue
Cincinnati, OH 45239

Cleveland Clinic Foundation
Medical Technologist Program
One Clinic Center (L11)
9500 Euclid Avenue
Cleveland, OH 44195-5130

Cleveland Metropolitan General
Hospital
Medical Technologist Program
3395 Scranton Road
Cleveland, OH 44109

Fairview General Hospital
Medical Technologist Program
18101 Lorain Avenue
Cleveland, OH 44111-5656

St. Alexis Hospital
Medical Technologist Program
5163 Broadway Avenue
Cleveland, OH 44127

University Hospitals of Cleveland
Medical Technologist Program
2074 Abington Road
Cleveland, OH 44106

Ohio State University
Medical Technologist Program
1583 Perry Street
Columbus, OH 43210

Good Samaritan Hospital and Health
Center
Medical Technologist Program
2222 Philadelphia Drive
Dayton, OH 45406

St. Elizabeth Medical Center
Medical Technologist Program
601 Edwin C. Moses Boulevard
Dayton, OH 45408

Wright State University
Medical Technologist Program
235 Biology Sciences Building
Dayton, OH 45401

Kettering College of Medical Arts
Medical Technologist Program
3535 Southern Boulevard
Kettering, OH 45429

Southwest General Hospital
Medical Technologist Program
18697 East Bagley Road
Middleburg Heights, OH 44130

St. Charles Hospital
Medical Technologist Program
2600 Navarre Avenue
Oregon, OH 43616-3297

Ohio Valley Hospital
Medical Technologist Program
1 Ross Park Boulevard
Steubenville, OH 43952

Mercy Hospital
Medical Technologist Program
2200 Jefferson Avenue
Toledo, OH 43624

Riverside Hospital
Medical Technologist Program
1600 North Superior Street
Toledo, OH 43604

Trumbull Memorial Hospital
Medical Technologist Program
1350 East Market Street
Warren, OH 44482

St. Elizabeth Hospital Medical Center
Medical Technologist Program
1044 Belmont Avenue
Youngstown, OH 44501-1790

Western Reserve Care System
Medical Technologist Program
500 Gypsy Lane
Youngstown, OH 44502

Oklahoma

Valley View Regional Hospital
Medical Technologist Program
430 North Monte Vista
Ada, OK 74820

St. Mary's Hospital
Medical Technologist Program
305 South Fifth Street
Enid, OK 73702-0232

Comanche County Memorial Hospital
Medical Technologist Program
P.O. Box 129
Lawton, OK 73502

Muskogee Regional Medical Center
Medical Technologist Program
300 Rockefeller Drive
Muskogee, OK 74401

Mercy Health Center
Medical Technologist Program
4300 West Memorial Road
Oklahoma City, OK 73120

St. Anthony Hospital
Medical Technologist Program
1000 North Lee Street, Box 205
Oklahoma City, OK 73101

University of Oklahoma at Oklahoma
    City
Medical Technologist Program
P.O. Box 26901
Oklahoma City, OK 73190

St. Francis Hospital
Medical Technologist Program
6161 South Yale Avenue
Tulsa, OK 74136

Oregon

Oregon Institute of Technology
Medical Technologist Program
3201 Campus Drive
Klamath Falls, OR 97601-8801

Oregon Health Sciences University
Medical Technologist Program
3181 Southwest Sam Jackson Park
Portland, OR 97201

Pennsylvania

Abington Memorial Hospital
Medical Technologist Program
1200 Old York Road
Abington, PA 19001

Allentown Hospital
Medical Technologist Program
17th and Chew Street
Allentown, PA 18201

Sacred Heart Hospital
Medical Technologist Program
421 Chew Street
Allentown, PA 18201

Altoona Hospital
Medical Technologist Program
7th Street and Howard Avenue
Altoona, PA 16603

Neumann College
Medical Technologist Program
Convent Road
Aston, PA 19014

St. Luke's Hospital
Medical Technologist Program
801 Ostrum Street
Bethlehem, PA 18015

The Bryn Mawr Hospital
Medical Technologist Program
130 South Bryn Mawr Avenue
Bryn Mawr, PA 19010

Geisinger Medical Center
Medical Technologist Program
North Academy Avenue
Danville, PA 17822

Rolling Hill Hospital
Medical Technologist Program
60 East Township Line Road
Elkins Park, PA 19117

Saint Vincent Health Center
Medical Technologist Program
232 West 25th Street
Erie, PA 16544

Harrisburg Hospital
Medical Technologist Program
South Front Street
Harrisburg, PA 17101

Polyclinic Medical Center
Medical Technologist Program
2601 North 3rd Street
Harrisburg, PA 17110

Conemaugh Valley Memorial Hospital
Medical Technologist Program
1086 Franklin Street
Johnstown, PA 15905-4398

Lancaster General Hospital
Medical Technologist Program
555 North Duke Street
Lancaster, PA 17603

St. Joseph Hospital and Health Care
Center
Medical Technologist Program
250 College Avenue, Box 3509
Lancaster, PA 17604

Latrobe Area Hospital
Medical Technologist Program
West 2nd Avenue
Latrobe, PA 15650

McKeesport Hospital
Medical Technologist Program
1500 Fifth Avenue
McKeesport, PA 15132

Hahnemann University Hospital
Medical Technologist Program
Broad and Vine Streets, MS 505
Philadelphia, PA 19102

Lankenau Hospital
Medical Technologist Program
Lancaster and City Line Avenue
Philadelphia, PA 19151

Nazareth Hospital
Medical Technologist Program
2601 Holme Avenue
Philadelphia, PA 19152

Pennsylvania Hospital
Medical Technologist Program
8th and Spruce Streets
Philadelphia, PA 19107

Temple University
Medical Technologist Program
3307 North Broad Street
Philadelphia, PA 19140

Thomas Jefferson University
Medical Technologist Program
130 South 9th Street, Room 1924
Philadelphia, PA 19107-5770

Allegheny General Hospital
Medical Technologist Program
320 East North Avenue
Pittsburgh, PA 15212-9986

University of Pittsburgh
Department of Medical Technology
209 Pennsylvania Hall
Pittsburgh, PA 15261

Western Pennsylvania Hospital
Medical Technologist Program
4900 Friendship Avenue
Pittsburgh, PA 15224

Reading Hospital and Medical Center
Medical Technologist Program
6th and Spruce Streets
Reading, PA 19603

St. Joseph Hospital
Medical Technologist Program
12th and Walnut Streets, Box 316
Reading, PA 19603

Robert Packer Hospital
Medical Technologist Program
Guthrie Square
Sayre, PA 18840

Scranton Medical Technology
Consortium
Medical Technologist Program
700 Quincy Avenue
Scranton, PA 18510

Washington Hospital
Medical Technologist Program
155 Wilson Avenue
Washington, PA 15301

Chester County Hospital
Medical Technologist Program
701 East Marshall
West Chester, PA 19380

Wilkes Barre General Hospital
Medical Technologist Program
North River and Auburn Streets
Wilkes-Barre, PA 18764

Divine Providence Hospital
Medical Technologist Program
1100 Grampian Boulevard
Williamsport, PA 17701

York Hospital
Medical Technologist Program
1001 South George Street
York, PA 17405

Puerto Rico

Interamerican University-Metro
Campus
Metropolitan Campus
Medical Technologist Program
P.O. Box 1293
Hato Rey, PR 00919-1293

Catholic University of Puerto Rico
Medical Technologist Program
P.O. Station Number 6
Ponce, PR 00732

Interamerican University-San German
Medical Technologist Program
Call Box 5100
San German, PR 00753

University of Puerto Rico
Medical Technologist Program
GPO Box 5067
San Juan, PR 00936

University of the Sacred Heart
Medical Technologist Program
POB 1283, Loiza Station
Santurce, PR 00914

Rhode Island

General Hospital, Rhode Island
Medical Center
Medical Technologist Program
P.O. Box 8269
Cranston, RI 02920

St. Joseph Hospital OLF Unit
Medical Technologist Program
200 High Service Avenue
North Providence, RI 02904

Memorial Hospital of Rhode Island
Medical Technologist Program
111 West Brewster Street
Pawtucket, RI 02860

Rhode Island Hospital
Medical Technologist Program
593 Eddy Street
Providence, RI 02902

South Carolina

Anderson Memorial Hospital
Medical Technologist Program
800 North Fant Street
Anderson, SC 29621

Medical University of South Carolina
College Health Related Professions
Medical Technology Education
Department
171 Ashley Avenue
Charleston, SC 29425

Baptist Medical Center at Columbia
Medical Technologist Program
Taylor at Marion
Columbia, SC 29220

McLeod Regional Medical Center
Medical Technologist Program
555 East Cheves Street
Florence, SC 29501

South Dakota

St. Luke's Hospital-Midland Regional
Medical Center
Medical Technologist Program
305 South State Street
Aberdeen, SD 57401

Rapid City Regional Hospital
Medical Technologist Program
353 Fairmont Boulevard
Rapid City, SD 57701

Sioux Valley Hospital
Medical Technologist Program
1100 South Euclid Avenue
Sioux Falls, SD 57117-5039

Sacred Heart Hospital
Mt. Marty College
Medical Technologist Program
1106 West Eighth
Yankton, SD 57078

Tennessee

Austin Peay State University
Medical Technologist Program
Clarksville, TN 37044

Lincoln Memorial University
Medical Technologist Program
Harrogate, TN 37752-0901

Holston Valley Hospital and Medical
Center
Medical Technologist Program
West Ravine Road
Kingsport, TN 37662

University of Tennessee Medical
Center at Knoxville
Medical Technologist Program
1924 Alcoa Highway
Knoxville, TN 37920

St. Francis Hospital
Medical Technologist Program
5959 Park Avenue
Memphis, TN 38119-5150

University of Tennessee Memphis
Medical Technologist Program
847 Monroe Avenue, Room 431
Memphis, TN 38163

St. Thomas Hospital
Medical Technologist Program
P.O. Box 380, 4220 Harding
Nashville, TN 37202

Tennessee State University
Meharry Medical College
Medical Technologist Program
School of Medical Technology
3500 John A. Merritt Boulevard
Nashville, TN 37203

Vanderbilt University Medical Center
Medical Technologist Program
402 Oxford House
Nashville, TN 37212

Texas

Hendrick Medical Center
Medical Technologist Program
1242 North 19th
Abilene, TX 79601-2316

Northwest Texas Hospital
Medical Technologist Program
1501 Coulter
Amarillo, TX 79106

St. Anthony's Hospital
Medical Technologist Program
P.O. Box 950
Amarillo, TX 79176

Austin State Hospital
Medical Technologist Program
4110 Guadalupe Street
Austin, TX 78751

St. Elizabeth Hospital
Medical Technologist Program
2830 Calder Avenue
Beaumont, TX 77726-5405

Robert L. Thompson Strategic
Hospital
Medical Technologist Program
School of Medical Technology
Carswell AFB, TX 76127

Corpus Christi State University
Medical Technologist Program
6300 Ocean Drive
Corpus Christi, TX 78412

University of Texas Southwestern
Medical Center
Southwest Allied Health Sciences
School
Medical Technologist Program
5323 Harry Hines Boulevard
Dallas, TX 75235

Pan American University
Medical Technologist Program
1201 West University Drive
Edinburg, TX 78539

University of Texas at El Paso
Medical Technologist Program
1101 North Campbell
El Paso, TX 79968

Harris Methodist Fort Worth
Medical Technologist Program
1301 Pennsylvania
Fort Worth, TX 76104

Tarleton State University
Medical Technologist Program
1625 West Myrtle
Fort Worth, TX 76104

University of Texas Medical Branch
School of Allied Health Sciences
Medical Technologist Program
J-28 Room 4-442
Galveston, TX 77550

Harris County Hospital District
Ben Taub Hospital
Medical Technologist Program
1502 Taub Loop
Houston, TX 77030

Methodist Hospital
Medical Technologist Program
6565 Fannin Mall Street 205
Houston, TX 77030

St. Luke's Episcopal Hospital
Medical Technologist Program
6720 Bertner Avenue
Houston, TX 77030

Texas Southern University
Medical Technologist Program
3100 Cleburne
Houston, TX 77004

University of Texas Health Sciences
Center at Houston
Medical Technologist Program
P.O. Box 20708
Houston, TX 77225

University of Houston-Clearlake
Medical Technologist Program
2700 Bay Area Boulevard
Houston, TX 77058-1098

Texas Technical University Health
Sciences Center
Medical Technologist Program
School of Allied Health
Lubbock, TX 79430

Midland Memorial Hospital
Medical Technologist Program
2200 West Illinois Street
Midland, TX 79701

Shannon West Texas Memorial
Hospital
Medical Technologist Program
120 East Harris, P.O. Box 1879
San Angelo, TX 76902

Baptist Memorial Hospital System
Medical Technologist Program
111 Dallas Street
San Antonio, TX 78286

University of Texas Health Sciences
Center at San Antonio
Medical Technologist Program
7703 Floyd Curl Drive
San Antonio, TX 78284

Southwest Texas State University
Program in Clinical Lab Sciences
San Marcos, TX 78666-4616

Wadley Regional Medical Center
Medical Technologist Program
1000 Pine Street
Texarkana, TX 75501

University of Texas at Tyler
Medical Technologist Program
3900 University Boulevard
Tyler, TX 75701

Wichita General Hospital
Medical Technologist Program
1600 8th Street
Wichita Falls, TX 78307

Utah

McKay Dee Hospital Center
Medical Technologist Program
3939 Harrison Boulevard
Ogden, UT 84409

Weber State College
Medical Technologist Program
3750 Harrison Boulevard
Ogden, UT 84408-3905

Brigham Young University
Medical Technologist Program
761 WIDB
Provo, UT 84602

University of Utah
Medical Technologist Program
27 Skaggs Hall
Salt Lake City, UT 84112

Vermont

University of Vermont
Medical Technologist Program
302 Rowell Building
Burlington, VT 05405

Virginia

University of Virginia Medical Center
Medical Technologist Program
Box 268-Medical Center
Charlottesville, VA 22908

Memorial Hospital
Medical Technologist Program
142 South Main Street
Danville, VA 24541

Fairfax Hospital
Medical Technologist Program
3300 Gallows Road
Falls Church, VA 22046

Rockingham Memorial Hospital
Medical Technologist Program
235 Cantrell Avenue
Harrisonburg, VA 22801

Norfolk State University
Medical Technologist Program
2401 Corprew Avenue
Norfolk, VA 23504

Old Dominion University
Medical Technologists Program
School of Medical Laboratory
Sciences
Old Science 209
Norfolk, VA 23529

Medical College of VA/Virginia
Commonwealth University
Medical Technologist Program
MVC Station-Box 583
Richmond, VA 23298

Carilion Health Systems
Roanoke Memorial Hospital
Medical Technologist Program
Belleview at Jefferson
Roanoke, VA 24033

King's Daughters' Hospital
Medical Technologist Program
P.O. Box 3000
1410 North Augusta Street
Staunton, VA 24401

Washington

St. John's Medical Center
Medical Technologist Program
1614 East Kessler Boulevard
Longview, WA 98632

Children's Hospital and Medical
Center
Medical Technologist Program
4800 Sand Point Way, NE
Seattle, WA 98105

Laboratory of Pathology of Seattle
Medical Technologist Program
1229 Madison #500
P.O. Box 14950
Seattle, WA 98114-0950

University of Washington
Medical Technologist Program
Department of Laboratory
Medicine SB-10
Seattle, WA 98195

Deaconess Medical Center
Medical Technologist Program
800 West Fifth Avenue
Spokane, WA 99210

Sacred Heart Medical Center
Medical Technologist Program
West 101 Eighth Avenue, TAF-C9
Spokane, WA 99220

Tacoma General Hospital
Medical Technologist Program
315 South K Street, P.O. Box 5277
Tacoma, WA 98405

Central Washington University
Medical Technologist Program
1114 West Spruce, Suite 34
Yakima, WA 98902

West Virginia

West Virginia University
Medical Technologist Program
2138 Basic Sciences Building
Morgantown, WV 26506

West Liberty State College
Medical Technologist Program
Department of Medical Technology
West Liberty, WV 26074

Wisconsin

St. Elizabeth Hospital
Medical Technologist Program
1506 South Oneida Street
Appleton, WI 54915

Sacred Heart Hospital
Medical Technologist Program
900 Clairemont Avenue
Eau Claire, WI 54701

St. Vincent Hospital
Medical Technologist Program
P.O. Box 13508
Green Bay, WI 54307

University of Wisconsin-Madison
Medical Technologist Program
1300 University, 6175 MSC
Madison, WI 53706

St. Joseph's Hospital
Medical Technologist Program
611 St. Joseph Avenue
Marshfield, WI 54449

Clement J. Zablocki VA Medical
Center
Medical Technologist Program
5000 West National Avenue
Milwaukee, WI 53295

Milwaukee County Medical Complex
Medical Technologist Program
8700 West Wisconsin Avenue
Milwaukee, WI 53226

Sinai Samaritan Medical Center
Medical Technologist Program
Mount Sinai Campus
950 North 12th Street
P.O. Box 342
Milwaukee, WI 53201

St. Mary's Hospital
Medical Technologist Program
2323 North Lake Drive
P.O. Box 503
Milwaukee, WI 53201

University of Wisconsin-Milwaukee
School of Allied Health Professions
Medical Technologist Program
P.O. Box 413
Milwaukee, WI 53201

St. Luke's Memorial Hospital
Medical Technologist Program
1320 South Wisconsin Avenue
Racine, WI 53403

Waukesha Memorial Hospital
Medical Technologist Program
725 American Avenue
Waukesha, WI 53186

Wausau Hospital Center
Medical Technologist Program
333 Pine Ridge Boulevard
Wausau, WI 54401

West Allis Memorial Hospital
Medical Technologist Program
8901 West Lincoln Avenue
West Allis, WI 53227

Wyoming

University of Wyoming
Medical Technologist Program
P.O. Box 3837 University Station
Laramie, WY 82071

THE SCOPE OF PRACTICE OF THE CLINICAL LABORATORY SCIENCES

The "Scope of Practice" describes in general terms the services provided by clinical laboratory scientists. Clinical laboratory personnel, as members of the health care team, are responsible for:

1. Assuring reliable test results which contribute to the prevention, diagnosis, prognosis, and treatment of physiological and pathological conditions. This assurance requires:

   A. Producing accurate test results.
   B. Correlating and interpreting test data.
   C. Assessing and improving existing laboratory test methods.
   D. Designing, evaluating, and implementing new methods.

2. Designing and implementing cost-effective administrative procedures for laboratories, including their services and personnel.

3. Designing, implementing, and evaluating processes for education and continued education of laboratory personnel.

4. Developing and monitoring a Quality Assurance System to include:

   A. Quality control of services.
   B. Competence assurance of personnel.

5. Promoting an awareness and understanding of the services they render to the consumer/public and other health care professionals.

Source: Fiorella, B. J., and A. Maturen. "Statements of Competence for Practitioners in the Clinical Laboratory Sciences," *American Journal of Medical Technology*, vol. 47, no. 8, August 1981, p. 649.

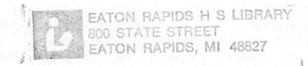

BIBLIOGRAPHY

Allied Health Education Directory, 1989. 17th ed. Division of Allied Health Education and Accreditation. Chicago: AMA, 1989.

Allied Health Services: Avoiding Crises: Report of a Study. Division of Health Care Services, Institute of Medicine, National Academy of Sciences. Washington, D.C.: National Academy Press, June 1988.

Bailey, Richard M. *Clinical Laboratories and the Practice of Medicine.* Berkeley: McCutchan Publishing Co., 1979.

Benezra, Nat. "Laboratory Salaries and Benefits: Are They Keeping Pace?" Part one, special report. *Medical Laboratory Observer* (January 1987): 30–34.

Benezra, Nat. "Laboratory Salaries and Benefits: Dissatisfaction in the Ranks." Part two, special report. *Medical Laboratory Observer* (January 1987): 37–39.

Castleberry, B. M., A. M. Kuby, and B. E. Bryant. "Wages and Vacancy Survey of Medical Laboratory Positions in 1988," parts 1 and 2. *Laboratory Medicine* (May-June 1989): 332–336; 437–441.

Fiorella, Beverly J. and Andrew J. Maturen. "Statements of Competence for Practitioners in the Clinical Laboratory Sciences." *American Journal of Medical Technology*, 47, no. 8 (1981): 647–652.

"Future Directions of Clinical Laboratory Science Education Programs." Position paper. Washington, D.C.: American Society for Medical Technology, June 1987.

Godolphin, William. "Robotics: Boon or Bust in the Lab?" *Medical Laboratory Observer* (November 1988): 28–32.

Gossel, Thomas A. "Home Testing Products for Self-monitoring." *American Journal of Hospital Pharmacy,* 45 (May 1988): 1119–1126.

Herrick, Vivian. "The Heritage of the Clinical Laboratory." *American Journal of Medical Technology* 3:53–59 (1937).

"Independent Practice." White paper. Washington, D.C.: American Society for Medical Technology, 1987.

Karni, K., K. Viskochil, and P. Amos. *Clinical Laboratory Management: A Guide for Clinical Laboratory Scientists.* Boston: Little, Brown and Co., 1982.

Lifshitz, Mark S. and Robert P. De Cresce. "The Clinical Lab of the Future." *Medical Laboratory Observer,* 20, no. 1 (January 1988): 30–33.

"Medical Technology." *Occupational Outlook Handbook.* Bureau of Labor Statistics, U.S. Department of Labor. Washington D.C.: U.S. Government Printing Office, 1988.

Paxton, Ann. " 'Help Wanted' in the Clinical Laboratory: How Crippling are the Personnel Shortages?" *National Intelligence Report for Clinical Laboratories and Blood Banks,* 10, no. 7 (January 26, 1989), special insert.

Price, Glenda, editor. "The American Society for Medical Technology: A Short History." Houston: American Society for Medical Technology, 1982.

Price, Glenda. "Introduction." *Shaping the Future of Clinical Laboratory Practice: Proceedings of the Conference.* Washington, D.C.: American Society for Medical Technology, 1986.

Quality Assurance in Physician Office Laboratories: The Setting, the Issues, and Federal, State and Private Approaches, 3rd printing. White paper. Washington, D.C.: American Society for Medical Technology, May 1987.

Vaughan, Victor C. *A Doctor's Memories.* Indianapolis: Bobbs Merrill, 1926.

White, William D. *Public Health and Private Gain: The Economics of Licensing Clinical Laboratory Personnel.* Chicago: Maaroufa Press, Inc., 1979.

Williams, M. Ruth. *An Introduction to the Profession of Medical Technology.* Philadelphia: Lea & Febiger, 1971.

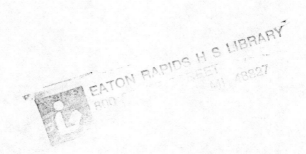

VGM CAREER BOOKS

OPPORTUNITIES IN

*Available in both
paperback and hardbound
editions*

Accounting Careers
Acting Careers
Advertising Careers
Agriculture Careers
Airline Careers
Animal and Pet Care
Appraising Valuation Science
Architecture
Automotive Service
Banking
Beauty Culture
Biological Sciences
Biotechnology Careers
Book Publishing Careers
Broadcasting Careers
Building Construction Trades
Business Communication Careers
Business Management
Cable Television
Carpentry Careers
Chemical Engineering
Chemistry Careers
Child Care Careers
Chiropractic Health Care
Civil Engineering Careers
Commercial Art and Graphic
  Design
Computer Aided Design
  and Computer Aided Mfg.
Computer Maintenance Careers
Computer Science Careers
Counseling & Development
Crafts Careers
Dance
Data Processing Careers
Dental Care
Drafting Careers
Electrical Trades
Electronic and Electrical
  Engineering
Energy Careers
Engineering Technology Careers
Environmental Careers
Fashion Careers
Fast Food Careers
Federal Government Careers
Film Careers
Financial Careers
Fire Protection Services
Fitness Careers
Food Services
Foreign Language Careers
Forestry Careers
Gerontology Careers
Government Service
Graphic Communications
Health and
  Medical Careers
High Tech Careers
Home Economics Careers
Hospital Administration
Hotel & Motel Management
Human Resources Management
  Careers

Industrial Design
Insurance Careers
Interior Design
International Business
Journalism Careers
Landscape Architecture
Laser Technology
Law Careers
Law Enforcement and
  Criminal Justice
Library and Information
  Science
Machine Trades
Magazine Publishing Careers
Management
Marine & Maritime Careers
Marketing Careers
Materials Science
Mechanical Engineering
Medical Technology Careers
Microelectronics
Military Careers
Modeling Careers
Music Careers
Newspaper Publishing
  Careers
Nursing Careers
Nutrition Careers
Occupational Therapy
  Careers
Office Occupations
Opticianry
Optometry
Packaging Science
Paralegal Careers
Paramedical Careers
Part-time & Summer Jobs
Petroleum Careers
Pharmacy Careers
Photography
Physical Therapy Careers
Plumbing & Pipe Fitting
Podiatric Medicine
Printing Careers
Property Management
  Careers
Psychiatry
Psychology
Public Health Careers
Public Relations Careers
Purchasing Careers
Real Estate
Recreation and Leisure
Refrigeration and Air
  Conditioning Trades
Religious Service
Restaurant Careers
Retailing
Robotics Careers
Sales Careers
Sales & Marketing
Secretarial Careers
Securities Industry
Social Science Careers
Social Work Careers
Speech-Language Pathology
  Careers
Sports & Athletics
Sports Medicine

State and Local Government
Teaching Careers
Technical Communications
Telecommunications
Television and Video Careers
Theatrical Design
  & Production
Transportation Careers
Travel Careers
Veterinary Medicine Careers
Vocational and Technical
  Careers
Word Processing
Writing Careers
Your Own Service Business

CAREERS IN

Accounting
Business
Communications
Computers
Education
Engineering
Health Care
Science

CAREER DIRECTORIES

Careers Encyclopedia
Occupational Outlook Handbook

CAREER PLANNING

Handbook of Business and
  Management Careers
Handbook of Scientific and
  Technical Careers
How to Get and Get Ahead
  On Your First Job
How to Get People to Do
  Things Your Way
How to Have a Winning
  Job Interview
How to Land a Better Job
How to Prepare for College
How to Run Your Own Home
  Business
How to Write a Winning
  Résumé
Joyce Lain Kennedy's Career Book
Life Plan
Planning Your Career Change
Planning Your Career of
  Tomorrow
Planning Your College
  Education
Planning Your Military Career
Planning Your Young Child's
  Education

SURVIVAL GUIDES

High School Survival Guide
College Survival Guide

VGM Career Horizons
a division of *NTC Publishing Group*
4255 West Touhy Avenue
Lincolnwood, Illinois 60646-1975